PEACE
AMONG THE
ANIMALS

PEACE AMONG THE ANIMALS

A Love Story of Hope, Loss, and the Zoo Within

ISABELLA ALLENA

TABLE OF CONTENTS

Prologue

I was fond of animals, even as a child, just something about them made me smile in no way a peer could ever.

There's a quote I relay to:

"Until one has loved an animal, a part of one's soul remains unawakened." ~ Anatole France.

In my perception, animals provided a sense of liberation from the pervasive presence of affliction and troubles that enveloped my surroundings. I harbored aspirations for my future, aspiring to pursue veterinary studies. Since childhood, I harbored a fervent passion for animal care, notwithstanding my hatred to the euthanasia aspect inherent in the job. I envisioned opening a practice of my own and uniting in matrimony with the individual I cherished most from my earliest years. Henry and I were childhood companions, our friendship enduring from grade school through high school. We attended prom together and cultivated numerous joint aspirations. During my high school years, I was the one meticulously crafting a life blueprint to lay out my trajectory for the approaching two decades.

We went to college together and were inseparable, dedicating so much time to studying and focusing on school that we overlooked the simple things in our relationship. Our marriage, entered into almost on a whim, succeeded by sheer luck. We skipped the typical honeymoon phase and went straight to work. Our honeymoon in the Galápagos Islands still involved working. My mom had wanted us to go to Paris, the city of love, but we opted for a more science-focused trip that turned into work. They say you never work a day in your life when you love your career, and we certainly did.

However, we spent so much time working and studying that we missed out on the essence of our relationship, which in turn, was cut short by the hardships of life. We planned meticulously without truly living in the moment. As my mother often reminded me, "Man plans, and God laughs," a once-amusing saying that became a harsh reality in my life. Our deep investment in our careers caused us to neglect the foundation of our marriage, proving that even the best-laid plans can fail when the heart's needs are ignored.

Chapter 1

A cheap starter in the Bronx was where I started my life. It was a lovely little home I could build with him. A small two-bedroom, two-bathroom brownstone with a small kitchen, and intimate living room, only 1000 Square feet. Despite being in a not-so-great area, we made it our home and quickly began to create a warm, loving environment.

I looked out the window to the children playing in the street; it just warmed my heart, they're so innocent and pure. I loved imagining my life with Henry as he unpacked our childhood homes in the living room.

Moving from Chicago, we only took the bare minimum since we couldn't spend an arm and a leg on shipping.

This was our first home together. Henry had lived alone for a while, but I had only lived out of my childhood home from college. Right after college, I married Henry, we moved for my schooling, and he got a job in the New York Public Schools as head of the Science department of a Middle School.

I received a degree from the University of Chicago in Biological Sciences with a focus on cellular and molecular biology and a minor in Latin. We moved to New York so I could continue my studies in veterinary school. I would always be incredibly grateful to Henry for uprooting his life for me. I dragged him across the country, made him recertify through New York, and restarted his life knowing no one but me.

So many people think that my husband is the brains of our relationship, but I was always the silent killer. Henry was a biology teacher, and we went to college together, both studying the sciences. We both loved to sit and read reports together, arguing about any flaws in the studies.

I helped him unpack as we both reminisced on all of our things. "Have I ever told you how much I love you?" I smiled

"Many times, and I love you at an amount no one else could ever compete with" Henry smiled

I pulled the old bird feeder out of the box, cleaned it up from the bird poop and rustiness that my father left on it. I hung it in the window, near where the children played. My dad gave me the feeder but no food, so I left it outside without food. Birds came and went, indifferent to the lack of grain.

Henry threw me onto the couch. The only furniture we had at the moment. "Good because you are not going anywhere, you are stuck for life!" He laughed

"I think I'm going to bake a cake for the tenants nextdoor." I said.

"That sounds sweet!" he yelled from the other room.

I brought out bundles of disorganized kitchen supplies "I think we may need to find the baking supplies first" I laughed

We had unpacked our basics and went on with our week. Henry had a job lined up at the middle school in Manhattan and I was a seamstress for the local boutique. Meanwhile, I was looking at veterinary schools which were far and few in-between.

I had a great track record from college, and I knew I wouldn't have a problem in school, I just needed to get in. Between school and trying to settle my life in a new state and city, I had my hands full of stress. I had to find new doctors, new insurance, new stores, new everything. I was starting my life from scratch, which was by far, no easy feat.

My mind was flooded from constantly worrying about my schooling, so I tried to distract myself from everything with baking which seemed to have turned out well. I didn't have any talents in baking or cooking so I was a little nervous about burning the house down. I knew no one so I hoped to make one friend, especially since we shared the same wall.

"Hi! My husband, Henry, and I recently moved in next door and wanted to bring a little warming gift" I smiled

"We'll hello, lovely to meet you, my name is Vera" She had a cigarette hanging out of her mouth and I immediately had preconceived notions.

I offered the cake hesitantly. She barely said a word and took the cake. I wished her a great evening. She closed the door on my face, and I headed back home. She had a very cold demeanor and seemed to be closed off to any new friends. I guess I expected more but I just couldn't find the words. I took the short two-step walk back to our door, a little shaken up by the cold aura Vera had given off.

~

The next day, Henry went to work, and I had the day to explore our new city. I wandered all day, looking for various places to settle as "locals". There was a small shop I went to that sold little tchotchkes to decorate the house with. I then went to a market to plan the next few days of meals. I tried to find organic, fresh produce to keep both myself and Henry in shape.

Later, I ended up at the local bar where I ran into Vera. She was drinking alone at the end of the bar, she seemed to have known the bartender. I always hated judging a book by its cover and I wanted so hard to get rid of that first impression of Vera.

"Are you catching yourself a new partner?" She said from across the bar

I was caught off guard by her blunt remarks "Excuse me?!"

"Why are you here if you are in a relationship" she asked confusingly

"I just have been wandering," I said blankly. I was trying to figure out why she was so invested in my relationship with my husband.

"And you wandered to a bar?" She joked

"I guess I did, I didn't know a bar was just for hooking up?" I said confidently

It was shallow to think that going to a bar meant you were single and looking to take someone home with you. I looked briefly at Vera's hand. No wedding ring made me think she was there for a man.

"What's your story?" she asked as she sipped her Scotch.

She seemed agitated that I was in a loving relationship I would never betray, or it was my presence. I felt a sense of loneliness radiate from her like she was used to not having anyone in her life.

"Well, I grew up in the suburbs of Chicago and recently moved here to Brooklyn with Henry who is a science department chair at a middle school in Manhattan and I am looking for a veterinary school," I explained

"Vet school? You're a girl, aren't you supposed to be looking at becoming a schoolteacher for your hubby?" She laughed, drunk from her bottomless glass.

"I always had a love for animals, and I wanted to make a living out of it" I wanted to stop the conversation since she seemed to have fit my idea of her perfectly.

"I like animals too, but you don't see me going out becoming a doctor," she said rudely

"Well, what do you do?" I asked expecting her to not be doing anything

"School secretary" she replied

"Well, that's nice!" I said.

 I finished my wine and threw my coat on.

"Not really but it's something" She ordered another round from the bartender. She didn't even need to say a word, yet the bartender knew exactly what she needed.

"I must be going it's getting late; I would love to get together with you and your?" Not wanting to make any assumptions, I stopped honestly not knowing.

"Oh, it's just me darlin'" she interrupted

"Well with you" I smiled as I began to walk out of the dimly lit bar, into the warm August evening.

 I got home to find Henry half asleep on the couch, I woke him from the heavy door slamming unintentionally and he scemed to have been surprised I came home so late. I was gone since he left for work this morning, so this was the first time we were seeing each other that day.

Coming out of a long lap after work. "Your home late, exploring town?" He said groggily

"Yes, I met our lovely neighbor again at the bar" I replied sarcastically

"The bar? Why were you there?" He asked me, knowing I don't drink often.

"I don't know I was just there," I said

"Well how is she, did you make a friend?" He added.

I explained how rude she was and how I didn't think it was a great idea to get involved with her. He assured me I was being dramatic, and New York was different from Chicago. I couldn't imagine staying here for long if everyone was going to be rude like that. Vera was a sad person who took her loneliness out on other people who were happy in life, it seemed.

She was the kind of person to take out her problems in the world. If the deli got her order wrong, she made it known. She made sure to let the worker know they ruined her day, despite not being very upset at all. Just the person to make someone's day even worse without a thought in the world.

I guess I had the vision of New York as this Broadway musical-style life with people who are living their lives to the fullest and have these amazing city jobs. How stupid was I...

Chapter 2

Henry and I were still settling into the new city life. We wanted to take in the New York experience together, so we decided to take as many opportunities as possible.

He came up to hug me from behind. "Hey, honey, I was thinking we should have a special date night to celebrate our move from Chicago. What do you say?"

As I stared at the birds in the window, I replied "That sounds like a fantastic idea! It's been quite a journey, and we deserve to treat ourselves. It's not like we have any food in the house anyway"

"I was thinking we could try that new Italian restaurant downtown. I heard they have amazing pasta dishes, and maybe we can get some gelato after?"

"That sounds perfect! I love Italian food and gelato!! Should we make a reservation for tonight?"

"I'll call and make a reservation for 7 o'clock. And maybe afterward, we can take a stroll through Central Park and enjoy the evening skyline of our new home."

"That sounds like a wonderful plan. I can't wait for our special date night. It'll be great to celebrate this new chapter in our lives together."

"Definitely!"

In a bustling corner of our new home, the aroma of garlic and tomatoes wafts from a cozy Italian restaurant. This was our first time going out in New York and we were excited for the fresh, new start.

Inside, cream tablecloths and dim lighting created an intimate ambiance. Others chattered animatedly, their laughter blending with the soft strains of Italian music.

Waiters bustled between tables, balancing trays of steaming pasta and fragrant pizzas. The clinking of glasses accompanied the symphony of flavors as diners savored each bite of homemade cuisine. Amidst the bustling atmosphere, the essence of Italy was palpable, transporting us to the bustling streets of Rome or the tranquil shores of Sicily with every savory bite.

Henry and I finally sat for dinner. I opted for a small portion of ravioli, while Henry indulged in a juicy steak. Later, we swung by a nearby creamery for some authentic Italian gelato.

To end the night, we walked through Central Park, watching the glistening sky full of stars. Each star is unique in its way, similar to how each path we take in life is unique. Each star holds a guide for us through the unknown, shaping our unique journey forward.

~

During college, I was so busy and never had time to go see doctors or plan my life post-college. Therefore, a lot of the appointments I was making in NY, were my first appointments like my gynecology appointments.

I was always a light sleeper, so if Henry was awake, I was awake. It wasn't ideal since I wasn't due to work until noon, but it was nice because I was able to see Henry off to work since he's always at work until late at night. He was usually a lot less stressed in the morning, so he was a pleasure to deal with. Henry was honestly a lot more mature which everyone picked up on.

"I have a doctor's appointment today and then I'm going to an interview in Manhattan," I explained.

"Well, we'll have to celebrate then!" he said enthusiastically.

"Celebrate what? I haven't even gone to the interview. It's also the first one of many so it's nothing to get excited about." I laughed.

Henry cuddled up on the couch with me. "Well, I know you'll get whatever the interview is for, so might as well plan early!"

I didn't think Henry understood the slim statistics of veterinary school acceptance. He went to school for teaching and got his masters in school administration in a dual program. I am in no way downplaying his job, but there are hundreds of school employees and not nearly as many vets.

"You're too optimistic!" I smiled.

Henry didn't fully realize how difficult vet school is to get into. "And you're too pessimistic!" he joked.

"Dinner tonight?" he asked.

"Sounds lovely, but no celebration until I know!!" I said.

"Fine..." he said hesitantly.

I went off to my appointments and Henry went off to work. I walked to the subway and took the train to midtown where I had a meeting with a tall powerful gentleman who was the deciding factor in my future dreams coming true.

Ultimately, I missed my doctor's appointment as I was so nervous, yet excited about my interview. I practiced what I would say all morning at Central Park to the birds chirping away at the bright blue sky.

I left Central Park in a hurry so I would not be late. Pushing everyone to the side, I hustled through the crowds to arrive early. I wanted to get a feel of the place, but I was not prepared for how large the science department alone was.

The sheer size of the city and the school was so overwhelming; I felt like I must have looked dumb as I wandered the building looking for where I was supposed to go while also getting distracted by the complexity of the different rooms.

I finally found the veterinary medicine front desk where I shuffled through all of my paperwork finding the name of the man, I was meeting. I think the woman at the desk could sense my fear and she assured me everything would be fine and that I had nothing to worry about. As I was casually speaking to her about Chicago, a man came out of his office in a fine Burberry suit which screamed class, to call me in.

He knew his secretary was from the Midwest as well. "So, tell me about yourself; what brings you to New York? I see that you're from Illinois." the interviewer asked curiously.

"Well, my husband and I just moved here for grad school. He is a science teacher downtown at the middle school and- I'm sorry, I am so excited to begin this new phase in my life." I said as I tried to contain myself.

"I grew up in Chicago and married my husband as we graduated from the University of Chicago. We are so excited to be here in the big city ready to take on the world!"

"You are just an eccentric little one, aren't ya?" he laughed.

"All 5 feet of me!" I smiled

He asked me why I decided to become a vet, I think he could sense I was nervous and wanted to ease my nerves.

"I have always loved animals ever since I was a child and I want to be able to help others keep their furry loved ones healthy. As a child, my father took us to an animal sanctuary in Ireland, just outside of Shannon, where I was so invested in watching the employees and doctors nurse these animals back to health. Anytime we were in Ireland, I lived on my grandparent's farm." I explained.

He continued to shuffle through my files. "Great! Looking over your resume, it is quite impressive, you seem to have been involved with animals all of your life," he said.

"Yes, I have been! I also have been volunteering at the local animal shelter since I was 12 years old, did work for my grandparents' farm, and spent my summers there in grade school. I learned a lot from them since they took care of all of the livestock themselves. In Ireland, having vets isn't the most common for farms so my grandparents did it all. I birthed my first calf at 9 years old!" I said.

"Wow impressive, I love your enthusiasm!" he smiled.

That interview was the most cliché interview I've been through, but it was exciting, nonetheless. Yes, I did live in Ireland for summers all through my childhood. Those summers in Ireland were some of the best I've had, and I will always treasure them. My grandparents loved to bring me out to the fields to ride horses and feed the pigs. They taught me all that I know about animals and fueled my desire to become a veterinarian.

My parents weren't very involved in my life so oftentimes they would ship me off to my grandparents in Ireland. While it wasn't ideal for a young child, I gained a lot of my knowledge from them.

I rushed home not even thinking about the appointment that I missed, I was so excited to tell Henry how much the school loved me.

"How did your interview go?" he asked.

I ran over to hug him. "Oh, it went fantastic Henry!" I said

"Does this call for celebration?" he asked excitedly

"Not yet, I still have a lot to go…" I paused.

"Well, I still think we can celebrate this little win." he smiled.

In the rare intimate moment we had, we both started in the living room and slowly made our way to the bedroom.

"Yea? How so?" I asked him with a big smile.

He began to kiss my neck and whispered in my ear "I can think of some ideas"

We melted into each other's arms, our kisses sparking an irresistible longing which guided us to the bedroom. With gentle hands, he undressed me, each touch sending waves of anticipation through my body. As he joined me, our connection deepened with every slow, deliberate movement. His touch on my breast sent tingles of pleasure coursing through me, heightening our shared ecstasy with each tender caress. Lost in the rhythm of our passion, our moans filled the room, echoing our complete surrender to each other.

Sex wasn't a huge priority in our lives, but when it happened, we threw ourselves into it completely. With both of us juggling hectic schedules, this intimate connection became a rare and cherished escape from the chaos of our daily routines. It was more than just physical release; it was a sanctuary where we could let go of our worries and simply be together, finding comfort and rejuvenation in each other's embrace.

Chapter 3

Remember that doctor's appointment I missed? Well, it ended up biting me in the butt. I really didn't think anything of it. I didn't see many doctors in college, and I never cared to in high school so I thought it would be best to finally get ahead of my health.

The office was oddly welcoming. It was very women-based, and it felt warm rather than the cold blank doctor's offices that were the norm at every other office out there. I checked in with a cheerful young lady who seemed excited to do her job.

I sat in the waiting room scrolling through my emails, not thinking of anything. I wanted to get it over with and get on with my day. I was quickly called back and met with another cheery employee who took care of my medical records, vitals, and any other information the doctor needed. I was handed a thin, paper gown that covered only my backside. I waited for the doctor to come in, holding my gown together trying to not rip it.

The doctor came in shortly after I had changed. She had a cheerful mood so early in the morning. I wasn't prepared for anything, so I felt very blind going in. I watched her prepare everything for the appointment. I wasn't too panicked, but I still felt nervous as my mind always goes to the worst possible situations.

She was quick to remind me of the appointment that I missed due to my interview. I distracted myself by telling her about my meeting with the Vet school. Invested in the conversation, she gave a sense of friendship like we had known each other for years. I told her I had a long way to go before knowing information about but we both shared excitement for my future.

The doctor began her exam. "Okay, so just lay back and try and relax; I'm going to start externally to see for any abnormalities in your ovaries and uterus."

"Are you and your husband sexually active?" She asked

"Yes, I would say once or twice every two weeks." I said

"Okay, do you have any pain or discomfort during sex?" She asked

"Nope" I lied knowing that I wasn't having the mind-blowing sex every newlywed would typically have, I ignored it because I knew we were both so busy launching our careers.

She continuously asked the basic questions and I mindlessly answered until the topic of pregnancy came up. I had wanted to have children all my life, but I knew I needed to wait so I could keep my timeline of vet school on track. Henry wanted children as well, but he's always busy with work too. Handling an entire school science department was not the easiest and he needed to make his mark within the school district.

"Are you trying to get pregnant?" she asked,

"I'm not trying to but I'm not, not trying." I explained, "Henry is working a lot and I'm working on my career, so I don't know if a child will be in the very near future, but I'd be willing to stop everything to have a baby."

"Good, so do you track your menstrual cycle to avoid sex, or do you do anything to avoid pregnancy?" she asked.

I didn't think of any red flags from my period "Not really, my period has been a bit more irregular, but I just thought it was because of our move and the stresses of life," I said

"Okay, so it was normal previously?" she asked in a slightly concerned tone.

"Yes, and in that time, I would track my period and Henry would pull out before," I explained, "I'm sorry, is that inappropriate?" I laughed.

"No, I'm here to get all of your information to make sure you're on the right track." she smiled.

Henry was a twin and had an older sister, and I was an only child. I knew genetics didn't work in our favor considering pregnancy wasn't easy in either of our families. I might have a more difficult time getting pregnant, but also if I were to get pregnant then I could have a chance of having twins.

"Okay, so I'm going to begin internally, you will feel a lot of pressure," she explained as she went in

I tried to reassure my self that everything was normal. "So, you think my period is due to stress too?" I asked

"It's very likely, periods are very sensitive when it comes to issues with stress like a career change or a big move, both of which you are doing." she reiterated.

My period was very straightforward, and I didn't think anything of having an issue with it. A lot of times my period would be late or come at a completely different time. I guess I didn't think much of it because Henry and I weren't trying to get pregnant or prevent a pregnancy.

"Your cervix looks good, I just want to do a quick swab, but nothing looks out of the ordinary," she said positively.

"I really need to use the bathroom, is that normal?" I asked, knowing that actually was not normal from my previous exams.

"The speculum is putting pressure on your bladder; I'm almost done and once I am you can use the bathroom," she assured me.

"You will have some slight spotting, but nothing out of the ordinary; it's just your cervix irritated by my swabs," she said as she finished up.

I felt the strong urge to go to the bathroom, but she wouldn't let me go. She didn't seem to be in a rush, yet still needed to get everything in at a time frame that fit her schedule. I was finally able to go to the bathroom and there was a lot of blood. It alarmed me a bit and I mentioned it to her, yet she dismissed it and gave me a pad.

At this time in my life, I thought I had a tiny, sensitive bladder but now looking back, I realized my bladder had bigger issues than being small.

"Has anyone talked to you about having very dense breast tissue?" she asked.

I was still confused. "I mean I guess my husband has; I don't even know what that means," I said

"Basically, your breasts are firmer than average, but it is most likely nothing to worry about," she assured me.

"Do you have any history of breast issues in your family?" she asked.

My anxiety festered in my stomach. "No, why?" I said nervously

"I'm just covering all of my bases." she said confidently.

"So, you do monthly self-breast exams?" she asked as if anyone truly does those.

"What are you not telling me?" I blurted out.

"You have a lump in your breast, but at your young age, it could be anything from a Fibroadenoma to a cyst. I'm sure there is nothing to worry about!" she said in a calm, relaxed tone.

I rushed up and grabbed my bra and top in a panic. "Are you sure? I'm 23 years old, I can't have cancer or anything!"

"No one said anything about cancer, we will do an ultrasound and a biopsy to rule out cancer. You are worrying for no reason" she attempted to calm me.

"And you know how?" I asked.

"My biochemistry bachelor's as well as my four years of medical school, and four years of gynecology residency." she assured me.

I cut her off. "Yea yea yea, but do I have cancer?"

"I don't know, let's not get ahead of ourselves. Just relax, again breast cancer in your twenties is rare. Go to the front and schedule a biopsy. I will get the ultrasound done today so we can look over those scans with the biopsy. Do not worry because there are so many explanations for a lump and cancer is highly treatable in this day and age." she explained.

"I don't even have kids yet, I want a family, what am I going to tell my husband, we just got married-" I said

I began to panic thinking how I could explain this to Henry, how could I tell him that I could possibly have cancer?

She grabbed my arm as I tried to rush off. "Stop, you are going to tear yourself apart if you keep the thought of cancer in your mind."

"What else am I supposed to think about?!" I said.

"Vet school, plus you just moved here! Explore a little!" she exclaimed.

I calmed down a little bit. "No, you're right, okay, so schedule that, and go from there."

"Exactly, you will be okay." she hugged me as we walked to the front desk

"Oh, and Philomena!" she yelled before going back to work,

"DO NOT RESEARCH!" she stated to me

I stared blankly at her as I walked to the front knowing I would in fact stay up all night and research. I know that I don't have any clear diagnosis but knowing I had a lump made me feel sick to my stomach. Breast cancer didn't run in my family, I wasn't doing anything 'wrong', this all didn't make sense. After my mom passed from lung disease, I was always careful to stay away from cigarettes or pollution. I guess moving to New York City wasn't ideal. The constant traffic, the people lighting a smoke at every corner, these clear-cut carcinogens, but what's clear-cut about breast cancer?

~

I walked home slowly, not wanting to go home to see Henry. I wasn't sure how to explain to him something that wasn't even a fact yet. The pit in my gut grew larger as I got closer to home. I walked through the door with a cold, blank emotion on my face.

"What's on your mind?" Henry asked as he finished up dinner.

"Nothing, I'm just distracted with all of my paperwork due for vet school." I pulled an excuse from the top of my mind.

"You sure? I don't think *WebMD* has an animal tab."

He peered over my shoulder, as I smelled his garlic breath from the sandwich he had for dinner. Ignoring it, I pushed him away and tried to get him off my back so he wouldn't start thinking anything was wrong.

"Well, I'm comparing animals to humans, that's a class in vet school." I quickly changed the tab to drugs and supplements, comparing what animals could take and what people could take.

"Is it now?" he smiled, not thinking anything of it. He didn't seem to have a sense of concern.

"Yes, it helps us learn about the differences and similarities between animals and humans, did you know we are fairly similar? The only thing is, we have different placements of organs and stuff. Similar to drugs, there's a lot of drugs that animals and humans can take, but they will have such different effects." I explained.

He had no idea what I was talking about and probably didn't care "Got it, well I have to get up in the morning for a board meeting, we are trying to increase the budget for our spring musical.".

He kissed me. "Have a good night, love you."

"Love you too." I responded.

~

Later in the night, I decided to go out knowing my neighbor, Vera, would be at the bar yet again. I didn't want to talk to Henry about it because I wanted to be able to leave the conversation. I knew Henry wouldn't be able to just let go of it, but I knew Vera wouldn't harp on it or even care.

"You know it's not safe to be walking the streets alone at night. This isn't Kansas anymore." she laughed, clearly drunk.

"I'm from Illinois." I irritatingly responded

I contemplated if this was even a good idea. I didn't want to be beaten down by her attitude, but I also didn't want to be flooded with emotions from my husband.

She ordered another round "Oh... Well, same thing." she said

"Not really... anyway, I wanted your advice." I asked hesitantly

"It's 12:45 on a Friday night." She laughed

"Saturday morning." I corrected her

"We are not friends; we met a week ago and this is the second time you've talked to me." She replied

"I understand that, but I have no one and you're the first person I've met here." I responded in a desperate tone.

"I can't ever drink in peace." she sighed.

"Can you feel my breast?" I asked her bluntly

"Woah woah, I am not into that!" Came her quick.

"No, no, my doctor felt a lump in my breast, and I don't know what to do!" I replied

"Well, I'm not a doctor! Didn't your husband do something with medicine?" She said, waving down the bartender.

"My husband is a science teacher... besides I really don't want to talk to him about it" I said, "What do I do?!"

"Go home, it's too late and I am too drunk to deal with you." She said as she stumbled to the bathroom.

"Do you have a nice bone in your body!? I seem to always be a problem to you. I have no one here and all I want is someone to talk to." I argued

"Look, we are neighbors, you are also in your twenties, you don't have cancer, you're just being dramatic." She replied

I asked her, again, what her problem was. She paused, then ignored me again to go order another drink. I watched her signal to the bartender for one more and the check. Which he did with no problem. She paid her bill and walked away. I moved over to where she sat and looked at the check.

Four dirty martinis and three glasses of Jameson neat. A total of $82 with an $18 tip. A lot of money for a simple administrative assistant who lived alone in the middle of the Bronx.

Before I left, I sparked a conversation with the bartender who seemed to know a lot about Vera.

As I sipped my wine, I asked him "So, what's her story?"

"She didn't tell you?" He asked me in a sense of surprise.

"No?" I said, confused.

"Huh, well I'm not sure if I should tell you, not my business." He replied.

I could tell he wanted to tell me but didn't want to upset her or lose his best customer. There are two main professions people divulge all of their secrets to, a hairdresser and a bartender.

"No, I get it, but I want to know why she's so mean and miserable" I said

"Well, you didn't hear this from me" he said as he was polishing glasses. "Her ex-husband cheated on her, then ran away with this new lover who was 20 years younger than him. She then spiraled down the drain and began drinking"

"And you feed into her issues?" I asked him, laughing.

"Whatever pays the bills sweetie" he smiled, handing me my bill.

I left the bar and headed home. I thought about what the bartender told me, and it made sense why she was so miserable. Despite this, I think she could definitely turn her life around and help herself rather than drinking her sorrows away at some bar.

~

A week later I had a biopsy done. I wanted Henry to come with me, but once again, he had meetings at work that he could not get out of. I sat in the waiting room, alone, internally panicking from fear. I looked at everyone else in the waiting room. Some waiting for their first gynecological appointment, and some waiting to see their obstetrician for their ultrasounds.

There I was, waiting to find out the fate of my life. I will never forget the searing pain as the needle went into my breast. I had never had surgery or been in a position where I needed even a minor procedure done.

I felt the cold burn from the anesthetic and then the intense pressure of the large needle pulling little pieces of the lump out. I watched the doctor put the samples in a little cup, such a small amount for a large needle.

Henry didn't seem to think my lump was as big of a deal as I did. I wasn't sure if it was because he didn't want to worry me or because it really wasn't a big deal. Like everyone said, I'm in my twenties, how would I have cancer? There are so many different things it could be other than cancer, it could be a cyst, Hamartomas, or fibroadenomas. Cancer is the big thing that comes to mind.

I was frustrated by my husband's lack of empathy and his focus on work, but I guess we need the money. I walked home from the hospital without a thought in my mind except for this procedure. My emotions were as numb as my left breast.

All I had in my head was the stirring thoughts of the fact I could be cutting my time short. I went through the entire procedure like that, pondering my entire life thinking about what I wanted to do... All that could be cut short by some disease that doesn't even run in my family. After what felt like an hour's walk, I visited Henry at work.

Chapter 4

Sitting at the office, I realized Henry was busy and Vera was sitting at the front desk. I was so exhausted that the last thing I wanted to deal with was Vera's acerbic attitude.

"Hi, is Mr. Williams in?" I asked, staring at my phone.

"Yeah, he's in a meeting though," she said, as she looked up, "Phil? what are you doing here?"

"Visiting my husband, what are you doing here?" I asked annoyingly

"I work here," she said as equally annoyed

"You never told me that" I responded

"Never asked, I'm going out for a cigarette, Join in?" She asked

"No" I said bluntly

She dug through her purse for her lighter "Suit yourself, hubby will be out soon, just in a meeting for some kid who was smoking weed" Vera said

I stared at her as she became increasingly agitated from not finding her lighter. An awkward silence filled the room as I heard her digging through her purse and the parents arguing in the next room about their son.

Henry was a part of the discipline committee at the school which was needed as more children were becoming increasingly "unhinged".

"Marijuana, Mary Jane, gra-"

"Yea yea I got it"

I sat down to wait for Henry to come out of his meeting.

"I'll be outside Linda" she yelled as she walked to the courtyard

He walked some very angry parents and their tearful son out. "Hey sweetheart, how did your appointment go?" Henry asked

"Fine, so you never told me Vera worked here?" I asked him.

"Oh, yea she's just a paper pusher" he replied

Vera was an administrative assistant who never got her degree. I still wanted to know more about her and why she wouldn't open up to me. I hoped Henry would maybe get some information out of her.

I brought Henry lunch, despite knowing he had already eaten. He had another meeting with all of the science teachers about the year ahead, so I didn't have any time to talk with him about my procedure. Linda, the assistant principal, put the lunch in the fridge and walked me out. We had a brief conversation about how New York was treating me. I replied with how different it was and all of the different lives each person was living. She told me New York was a special place where each person was so different. She sent me on my way and headed back inside the school.

I walked to the subway to go home. I was sitting in the subway car, again panicking about my biopsy. I gripped my phone, thinking I would get a phone call any minute about my results. Despite my doctor saying it could take 2 to 4 days. I felt so alone like no one knew what was going on, even though no one actually knew what was going on. All were riding to their destinations, onto their divergent lives.

I understand how busy my husband's job is, I always remind myself he's got a massive middle school to handle and during the day I'm the least of his problems. It's something that I've dealt with. My mom was a teacher, and she was always involved more with her students than me. I remember sitting in her classroom waiting for her to get out of her "meetings" with other faculty.

In reality, she was sitting in the teacher's lounge, having a gossip session over cigarettes with other teachers. She was a life science teacher so that's where I learned a lot of my knowledge of plants and animals. Quite ironic since she died of lung disease caused by her smoking. I remember her always telling me to never smoke as she lit yet another one up.

~

My dad came over and I had a lot of questions for him regarding my health. My health was never a concern, and I didn't know much about my history. My dad didn't show any concerns nor did I, even after mom passed. We knew my mom's smoking caused her death so I never thought cancer would be a serious concern.

"Hey Dad, did mom smoke when she was pregnant with me?" I asked him as I pulled the wine out of the cabinet.

"Well good afternoon to you too sweetie" he said, settling himself on the couch

"Sorry. How are you doing?" I asked

"What's going on?"

He sensed something was wrong, ever since I was a kid I never got right to the point when it came to issues, I had. I didn't want to scare him without knowing for certain, so I lied.

"Nothing I just have to do a couple of intake forms for my new doctors" I responded

"Well, I don't think so, she didn't get into smoking until she had you" he said

Pondering if I was the reason she smoked

"Interesting..." I said

Obviously, I didn't cause my mother to smoke but the thought sat deep into my mind. My mom never wanted kids and made sure that I stayed an only child. She wasn't a mean person or abusive. She didn't want to be a mother or even try; she left all the parenting to my dad.

"I didn't mean it like that, she started when she went back to school, and I stayed home with you" he explained

"Oh, so it was work that got her hooked" I asked

My mind pondered to the thought ofHenry and how stressed he became with work. I prayed he didn't fall into the trap of smoking, follow down the mortal path my mother took. Especially through Vera's already solidified habit.

"I think so, she was working in a rough area but that's all that was available at the time" he continued

"Yeah, she stayed there for a while though. Why?" I asked

"She was a tough lady; she knew how to handle the delinquents" he said

He pulled Henry's whiskey out of the cabinet, declining my wine. Henry's vice was always whiskey which I didn't mind since it could've always been worse.

"I know now it's even worse now with drugs and gangs and kids growing up too fast, God bless Henry for doing what he does. It's probably why he needs this!" He said, nodding his glass.

"Yeah, he's definitely got his hands full" I replied

"How about lunch soon? You still haven't told me more about your interview. Oh! And before I leave, here's some mix for the bird feeder you stole from me" he added

I saw lunch as an opportunity to talk to him about my biopsy, but I didn't want to do it now because I didn't know anything concrete. Worrying him would make things worse, he already lost my mom, and I didn't want to worry him about possibly losing his only daughter.

My dad left, and I laid in bed thinking of all that could go wrong while realizing no one cares so why would I? I mean my husband is too wrapped up in work to even realize the gravity of the situation. My dad knows nothing about it because I refuse to tell him. Then I have no one else so why worry, right?

~

Henry came home soon after and found me lying in bed, researching yet again. He got changed and joined me in bed, leaning on me to read what I was searching for. Without saying a word, I could tell he was a little frustrated with me. He knew I shouldn't be researching and that all it was doing was making my anxiety worse.

He didn't want to read my 'propaganda', so he quickly got up to go get a snack. I stopped him by asking him different questions about cancer and reading him statistics from random websites.

"Did you know there are over 300k cases of breast cancer in the US?" I asked

"And did you know the survival rate is over 80% for most cases?" He replied "Besides, that counts both men and women, so you need to relax on the research"

"Every five minutes a woman will be diagnosed with breast cancer" I added.

Bringing a big bowl of snacks over he said, "Philomena, cut it out and eat some popcorn"

"Ugh, I can't stop… what if I have breast cancer?"
I replied

"And you may not! Therefore, you need to relax because it could be anything. There are other things it could be…that's not deadly." He said as he got comfortable in bed and turned the TV on.

Chapter 5

I had the longest week of my life while waiting for the doctor's call. Henry continuously tried to distract me without even mentioning my biopsy. It almost seemed like he forgot or didn't care. I couldn't think of anything else except for my breast. I continuously felt it and thought of every possible situation… nothing good.

~

Henry dragged me to a basketball game for his school to try and distract me. He could tell I was feeling down and anxious. He thought bringing me to his work events would keep my mind clear, but my anxiety was there to stay.

"It's the weekend, what do you need to go to work for?" I asked as I sat on my computer

"It's not work, just a basketball game" he responded

Henry and I argued as I didn't want to leave the house. He wanted to get me involved in his school, but I just didn't have the energy. I was exhausted from constantly worrying and researching.

He was by no means athletic, we never played anything in high school, and we never went to any games. Freshman year, his parents forced him into basketball. He was so bad they made him the team manager, another title for bench warmer and water bottle monitor.

He slammed my computer shut and threw my coat at me. He was excited to bring me, I wasn't too excited to go. I asked if Vera would be there, but he dismissed my question, trying to persuade me to like Vera. I couldn't see myself being friends with someone who constantly made it seem like I was a burden. Henry assured me that's just the way she is, nothing personal just her personality.

The minute I walked into the gymnasium; I saw Vera stumbling towards me. A drunk Vera was the last thing I wanted to deal with after the week I had been having. I prayed she would walk another direction, but she came right to my side.

She sat next to me, and she was the only one, I knew so part of me didn't really mind. "Hey, Phil! What're you doing here? This is a basketball game, not a zoo" she joked

"Very funny... I'm here supporting my husband!" I responded

"Oh, how sweet of you!" she said

I responded, tired of dealing with her attitude. "Look I know you don't like me, I'm not your type, but just because you're a part of the cool, popular group doesn't mean you can't be civil with me?"

"Ok ok relax, I'm laughing because you're here and your husband is not, yet again" she observed

"What do you mean he's right here!" I said before realizing he was missing. "What the heck..."

"Hell... We're grown-ups" she said, taking a sip of her water bottle that was definitely not water.

"Wait no look he's right there... See we are all good!"

I pointed to Henry who was sitting and talking with others who I did not know. I saw how quickly he made his own friends and quickly became accustomed to his brand-new life. All I had was a bitchy Vera, but Henry seemed to have many friends who liked him…he was popular.

"You panicked there a little, Phil" she laughed

"Stop calling me that, I'm not a 60-year-old single virgin" I argued

"What do you want me to call you?! Your names a million syllables" she claimed, laughing still

"Mena, that's what people call me" I stated

"Ok, I like Phil better. Phil" she said, "You ever hear from your orthodontist?"

"My what?" I asked her, becoming even more agitated

"Boobie doctor" she replied

"Oh no not yet. It's an oncologist by the way and technically he's not my doctor because I don't have cancer" I corrected her.

"Yet…" she said drunkenly

"Are you drunk?" I asked her

"For professional reasons, no" she responded

"Jeez Louise" I said, as I stood up to walk away

"I like you Phil" she laughed "You're like a puppy who's blinded by the world"

I kept trying to leave the conversation, but Vera kept taking shots at me. Instead of walking away, I continued to feed into her drunken pettiness.

"Is that how you see me?" I asked her

"Yes... You don't swear, you don't smoke, you don't drink" she responded

"I drink... Ugh anyway, I'm sorry I try to keep my world happy rather than dealing with all the problems in the world." I responded

"So blinded by the world..." she said

"I guess..." I pondered as I went to see Henry.

I know I am a child at heart, I love seeing the good in the world rather than pondering on all the ill-hearted acts that go on across the world. Why worry about war and bloodshed when you can just block it out to be happier in life?

It was hard to continuously be happy when everyone around you was so pessimistic. It was draining dealing with Vera constantly and watching my husband ignore the fact I could be dying. He seemed to ignore me the entire game, making me feel invisible.

Henry and I argued about how he acted like nothing was wrong. He claimed to have never even realized that he left me in the dust. As we stood in the lobby of the main office, we heard a scream from a distance. We ran over to see Vera standing on her desk panicking, refusing to leave. I saw the rat nibbling on a little piece of trail mix.

While I was figuring out a way to get the rat outside without harm, I listened to Henry argue with Vera about keeping food on the desk. I guess there was always a rodent problem. As soon as I leaned toward the rat, Henry yelled at me to get away from it. This scared the rat, and it ran into the closet.

Vera refused to get down and Henry ended up carrying her out of the office. I took an old paper box to the corner of the closet and managed to catch the rat within. Everyone watched as I ran the rat outside to the courtyard when Henry started yelling at me about different diseases rats carry. I knew the rat wouldn't hurt me, so I ignored him and walked away. Vera kept thanking me until I turned and screamed that she was the rat for being so rude, she was just a big bully who was miserable in life.

Henry grabbed me and we reluctantly went home. I gave up on constantly being the nice guy who let everyone walk all over her, but it was in my nature, it was so difficult to stand up for myself. To stop everyone from constantly running me around.

~

Henry and I sat at the kitchen table as we continued to argue about how he had been ignoring the reality of my health. I released my frustration on him, it felt so good to finally talk to someone about how I felt. I didn't sit and listen to others' problems while internalizing my own.

"Are you worried?" I asked him angrily

"About what?" he casually put his coat away, not thinking about what I'm asking; acting like any other day.

"Henry, I had a biopsy done on my breast and you barely said a word about it" I responded

"You and I are sometimes too similar," he said without answering me. "We internalize things without talking about them" he continued, "Trust me it's been eating me alive but it's not worth stressing out about when we just don't know yet."

"But there's a possibility" I said

"I know, I've thought of every possible outcome of this, and it distracts me every day. But I am trying to not get myself worked up about it because, again, we don't know. I distract myself with work to keep my mind busy" he added

I asked him "So, you care?"

"Of course, I care! How could I not?!" He replied

"You just seem to keep brushing it off" I said

"Yea... I know and I need to stop that, you're my wife and it's been extremely difficult to"

He hugged me as I began to sob. Anxiety consumed all of my thoughts and Henry began to sense that.

"Yeah, because I can't brush it off, I can't walk away from it, it's on me it's in my body." I replied

"When will you know?" He asked

"I don't know, hopefully within the next few days" I said

"Well, no news is good news" he said to me as we ate dinner.

Barely talking after our conversation. We both sat at the dinner table, our own thoughts the same, my possibility of cancer standing between me and a phone call.

~

The next day Henry left for work before I woke up. I went to the store to keep my mind off things. I ended up wandering and not buying anything because I couldn't calm my mind, my body felt hollow, but my brain was filled with all these different scenarios... Nothing good.

I kept Henry's words in my mind, that this could be anything. A simple benign lump which could be removed through a simple procedure. I remembered the doctor's words, telling me all of the different possibilities. All of which were a lot more common than breast cancer for my age.

While I was sitting in the coffee shop down the street when my phone began to ring. I anxiously searched through my purse despite knowing deep down who it was. My heart dropped as I read the caller ID as my doctor. I almost refused to answer it knowing it was a literal life-or-death situation. I paused, staring and holding the phone in my hands while having a deep feeling of dread to answer the phone.

Twenty-four years old and I listened to my doctor explain to me what triple negative breast cancer was and what that meant for me… A new cancer patient.

Chapter 6

Walking down the streets of New York, I decided to go make dinner for my husband. I bought fresh greens for a salad from the farmers' market on 4th Street. I, also, bought fresh pasta in Greenwich Village. Glass of wine after glass of wine, I made a creamy chicken Alfredo. Making sure my husband was ready for a scrumptious dinner so when he came home, I could tell him the wonderful news that I could have as little as six months to live.

Henry came home from a long day at work to me drunk off of a half bottle of Pinot Noir. As confused as he was, considering I rarely drank, he gladly sat for dinner. In order to cook Italian food, you must drink wine for it to be the best Italian food.

He began to shove down the pasta. "Did you hear from your doctor?" he asked

"I have six months to live!" I said in an ironically joyful tone.

He almost choked on a noodle as I casually dropped the horrific news.

"I know it's funny, me, the one who's always full of life, now has limited life, how ironic!" I laughed

"What did he say specifically" he asked in a concerned tone

"That I'm doomed" I replied

Henry grabbed the glass out of my hand before I spilled it on the new white carpet, "Okay let's put the wine down" he said while I pulled away.

I continued to fight him over going to bed. I just wanted to forget all that happened, and wine definitely helped.

He carried me to bed as I tried to seduce him for some dying sex. Henry left me waiting while he went to eat the rest of his dinner. He knew I'd pass out long before he came to bed. Despite my high alcohol consumption, I wasn't able to sleep because of all of my thoughts looming.

I was shaking from crying; I couldn't stop shivering because my anxiety was so high. I had never been close to death like this. The anxiety of my cancer diagnosis hit me like a tidal wave once I received the news. It was a whirlwind of emotions—shock, disbelief, and an overwhelming sense of vulnerability.

Suddenly, life divided into "before" and "after," and the weight of uncertainty became crushing. Every thought was tinged with fear, and my mind raced with questions about what the future held. It was a surreal experience as if I were standing on the cliff of an unknown abyss.

~

I woke up to my husband who was home from work for once. Hungover, I tried to ignore Henry's nagging to have a conversation about my diagnosis. I didn't want to have that conversation until I was ready.

The 'we'll get through this' and the 'you are so strong; you will beat' conversations. All the black-and-white conversations I wanted to skip. I just wanted to be alone, I wanted to lay in bed and cry.

Henry continued to try to pull information out of me and I kept telling him random facts I read on the internet. I didn't have a full workup or scans yet so, in reality, I knew nothing. Only that I had breast cancer, I didn't know the stage or if it spread. I guess it was nice to finally have Henry care.

I laid on the couch covered in blankets. "Are you going to work?" I asked

"No, I took the day off," he replied as he made breakfast and coffee.

Acting as though nothing happened. "Why? School needs you" I replied,

He put his computer down to finally talk without work distractions. "You need me" he stated

"I'm fine" I said

"No, you're not" he said

"Didn't realize you could tell my inner emotions" I argued

"What? - Never mind, just relax, we are going to get through this. Everyone has a time, and this is damn well not your time." he said, serving pancakes as I watched the birds in the window.

I wanted so badly to leave and go for a walk, but the heavy rain stopped me from my dramatic exit. Henry kept pushing questions as I ignored him. He slammed his phone down after I refused to tell him what the doctor said. He wouldn't let go and allow me to grieve in peace.

"So now you care?" I replied, tired of his tone

"What do you mean, I always cared" he claimed

"No, you didn't, you cared about your job but not me" I yelled as tears began to flow.

"Philomena, I needed to care about my job, who's going to pay the bills? I cared about you and still do. I just had no answers to what was going on so all I could do was sit and wait" he argued

I wanted to argue more and more but I felt so exhausted from fighting him and his work obsession. I understand that he needed to work and pay the bills, but I was drained.

I finally broke down, running to hug him. We couldn't understand why we were chosen to be tested like this. Obviously, no one should be put through this but why us. Out of the billions of people, not even, the millions in just New York, why me?

We stayed home the entire day, watching TV and cuddling up on the couch. This was the first day we were both at home together in a very long time... All it took was a cancer diagnosis. We love each other, we were just on different wavelengths. We both were so focused on our futures that we never took time to be in the present.

~

Henry went to work, and I sat at home digging through paperwork to find my old medical records and insurance information, all of which Henry handled for me. It took us some time since most of our important documents were packed away form our move.

I had a doctor's appointment to discuss my cancer in detail. I sat in the lobby looking around at all of the other people sitting. Thinking about how each person was there for the same reason but all completely different stories.

This was my first time in an oncology ward, so I had no idea how anything worked. Henry walked in at the last minute; this eased my anxiety a little to have him by my side.

It seemed as though he did his 3rd cancer talk of the day. Like he didn't care too much, it was a job to him. Granted it was a job to him, but he held my life in his hands, and I needed him to feel that way too.

"Good afternoon Mrs. Williams, how are you doing?" the doctor asked

Holding the gown together that left myself exposed to everyone in the room. "Could be better" I replied,

The doctor, nurse, and a medical student sat in the room with Henry and me as we were told the worst news of our lives. A doctor who had achieved my dream of having a medical degree, a nurse who was there to monitor, and a medical student who was just beginning his whole life… telling others who would be staring at the end of theirs.

"So, I want to start by discussing what we found in the biopsy and going more in-depth on what we had discussed on the phone" the doctor. began to explain

"Triple-negative breast cancer is an aggressive cancer, but we have options. We tested the cells within the tumor, and they tested negative for both estrogen and progesterone hormone as well as human epidermal growth factor receptor 2. Which is where we get the triple negative from. We are going to do a full-body MRI so we could see if the tumor metastasized anywhere else. The tumor is relatively small though, so I believe we caught it early." The doctor explained.

I remember my mind being so flooded with emotions that I failed to listen to the doctor's words. They all melted into one, the line between survival and death.

Both the doctor and student felt my breast like a learning tool, some 3D printed structure that wasused in medical school. The doctor discussed with the student where the tumor was located and what a malignant and benign tumor feels like. Just as I was sitting there pondering about staring death in the eyes.

Henry led the conversation regarding treatment and outcomes as I listened, thinking about what my future is to come. My survival rate was at 66%. I teared up as he explained my prognosis and how my age would work in my favor.

As he explained everything, he was feeling the tumor in my breast, I could feel the size just as he applied pressure. It was a hard lump like he could go in and pluck it out right there, such a weird feeling to have.

"Treatment-wise, I would like to start with surgery, and remove the tumor, I don't believe there's a need for a mastectomy because the tumor is small and you're young. I don't want to make a major change to your body so young. After a lumpectomy, we continue with chemotherapy to remove anything that was left behind." The doctor explained in a cold tone like he did this a thousand times.

"So, this is a confident solution?" Henry asked as he grabbed my shaking hand

"Yes, but we still need to look at the rest of your body to make sure nothing has spread because if it did spread, we are looking at a completely different treatment plan." He added

"And what would that entail?" I didn't even think about it spreading.

"It all depends on the location and size of the cancer. We would most likely go in with more aggressive chemo as well as radiation. But let's not jump to conclusions as we won't know until we see scans" he explained

The front desk scheduled a full MRI. Henry had to answer all of the questions because I couldn't clear my mind of all the dark thoughts swirling through my head. We also scheduled a lumpectomy for as soon as possible. We wanted to put this behind us and fight it head-on. I refused to put vet school in the past and I continuously prayed that it would never become a distant dream.

~

We went home and again lay in bed watching TV, not talking about what we had just discussed with the doctor. I don't know how I felt about it all or how Henry felt. We just sat there and acted like nothing happened.

After 6 episodes of Law and Order, Henry finally asked if I was okay. I looked at him with tears in my eyes and threw my head into his shoulder and cried. He comforted me as I let all of my emotions out that had been bottled up. I had no clue what I was going to do, all

I wanted to do was cry and lay in bed, closing the door to any conversation about cancer.

~

They managed to fit me in for an MRI the next day. A bright and early 6 am appointment after a sleepless night. I remember falling asleep to the music played on the noise-canceling headphones. It was the first sleep I got in over 24 hours. The noises of a loud machine faded out as the music slowly put me to sleep.

My MRI revealed a grim reality: a stage three diagnosis with tumors rampant throughout my reproductive organs, even invading my once-small bladder, which now struggled to function under the weight of its unwelcome guest.

The cancer had spread its web, entangling my chest wall and infiltrating my lymph nodes, leaving me melting in fear. With each image the doctor presented, it felt as though my world crumbled, the certainty of my life slipping away with every visible tumor on the scans. The sense of helplessness was suffocating as I grappled with the enormity of what lay ahead.

Chapter 7

Moving to a big city and being diagnosed with cancer straight away had its perks. Even less people I had to talk about it. Although, I hated it but since I had no friends, I didn't need to make the whole cancer announcement to anyone. I just had to tell my family home in Illinois, my boss, and Henry had to handle his half.

I walked into work to tell my boss I couldn't work anymore. I wasn't sure what he would think since they were already short staffed. Managing a small business that was basically a hole in the wall kind of place was a lot more difficult than it seemed.

My manager was a short tempered, corporate-style bully who could never do wrong. He seemed to always change the narrative, so he was in charge. I knew my cancer would be a dagger in his agenda. Not because he cared about my illness, just because he was losing a good employee who was able to produce a lot in a short time. It was always all about him.

Sewing was my one talent so I hoped that he would not completely destroy my confidence in it. The sicker I got the less motivation I had to work, the less ability I has to do tedious jobs like sewing. I couldn't do anything I loved, and I had to walk away to focus on my health rather than my happiness.

I walked into his office hesitantly, "good morning, Tom, can I speak with you?"

"Make it quick, you have to clock in, and we have a bridesmaid's consultation today!" He said, quickly going through his desk to get ready for the day.

"Yea about that... I have my formal resignation." I replied, "I have cancer"

"What do you mean? You look fine!" He replied angrily.

I was already annoyed by his lack of empathy.

"Yes, I know but I don't feel fine" I said

"This isn't a heavy labor, you just sit and sew, I don't see why you have to fully quit" he said

"Yes, but I can't do these tedious jobs like sewing and embroidering. I'm not saying I won't be back, but I need to, at least, take time off to focus on getting better" I explained

"Well… I can't guarantee a job if you decide to come back" he replied

"I understand… I don't think I will be back" I said

"Consider it because you're a good worker" he replied

"Yea…" he said

He almost reminded me of Vera, cold, self-centered, and narcissistic. I expected nothing less from him since he always feels the world revolves around him.

I left to go talk to Henry because his attitude through me for a loop. I hated when people were so rude for such unnecessary reasons. I knew Henry would cheer me up and have a great dinner ready.

"Hey how did it go at work?" Henry asked

"As good as it could have been" I replied

"That bad?" He laughed

"It's fine, I'm fine, he's just in his own little world." I said, "have you talked to your boss, yet?"

"I have not" he replied

"Why not? You need to talk to her about taking time off!" I exclaimed

"No, I know, and I will. I haven't had the time between her schedule and my schedule" he said

"Okay well find time because I am not going to these doctors' appointments alone" I said

"Okay, I will talk to her tomorrow, I promise!" He assured me

"Good, thank you!" I added, "Does Vera know?"

"I don't think so, if she knew the principal would know because Vera is a blabber mouth" he replied

"Well, my dad knows, does anyone in your family know?" I asked

"You're making it sound like were announcing a pregnancy" Henry laughed

"Henry…" I replied

"Okay, okay, most of my family knows, I called my brother after your initial appointment. My parents knew because my brother told them, and I have no clue if my sister knows." He explained

"Why don't you ever talk to your sister?" I asked, knowing I'd hit a nerve

"It's just not on the playing books right now" he said

"So, I'm dying and that still won't let you break that barrier between you guys" I replied

"I'll see her at the funeral" he argued

"Of course…" I said

Henry stopped talking to his sister when we were young, I never knew why, nor did he ever tell me. I assumed she moved out and they went their separate ways. But after multiple family gatherings on his side, I came to the conclusion that there was no relationship there anymore. It seemed like she was completely ostracized from the entire family. She didn't come to our wedding, but her husband and children came.

I stayed home to be alone and isolated myself from society. I couldn't deal with the content pity party from everyone after they find out I have cancer. It's crazy how people change so quickly once they see my illness.

~

Henry knew he had to finally talk with his boss about my diagnosis, but he felt the more he talked about it the more real it became. His boss was very understanding and sweet, very different from mine, so it wouldn't be a difficult conversation but still an emotional one.

"Good morning, Dr. Drew, how are you doing?"

'I'm doing well, thank you for asking" she replied, "I saw your text, what did you want to talk to me about?"

He sat down at the foot of her desk, "Well, its difficult to talk about but my wife was recently diagnosed with cancer, and I may need to take some days off, come in late, or leave early to help with her treatments" he explained

She stood up and hugged him tightly, "Henry, come here, let me give you a hug!" She said "I am so very sorry to hear this"

"Thank you, I hope you can understand if my work is affected" he replied

"Take all of the time you need! And please send my warmest wishes to Philomena, if you two need anything at all, let me know!" She replied, hugging him again

"Thank you, I truly appreciate it!" He said

Henry went to his office to work but his mind was filled with dark thoughts of losing his first love. With his stomach in knots, he was barely able eat anything or get any work done.

~

Every hour, Henry called me to see how I was doing, it was annoying, but I appreciated his concern. I hadn't started my treatments yet, so I wasn't sick or anything. I think he was more concerned with my mind spiraling down the drain than my physical health.

I was only emotionally exhausted because of the anxiety fueling in my body. The worst feeling was having an illness you couldn't control with a simple dosage of cough medicine or a bit of R&R. That's all I wanted, to go to the grocery store, pick up some cough syrup, take it to go to sleep and wake up all better, but that was far from possible.

While my downtime used to be going on a run through Central Park or shopping for new fabrics in downtown, I now stayed home and watched the birds feed in the window. I loved the birds because they reminded me of my life back home. My dad had a bird feeder when my mom became sick, and she would watch all of them while on hospice. My worst-case scenario was being in her shoes, and I knew I could very well be in that position soon. The birds symbolized life and strength. Even though my life quickly falling apart, I felt warmth in watching the bird fly around and live their lives like nothing could go wrong.

Henry came home after a long day's work, and he was exhausted so making dinner was not in the cards. He ordered food delivery and I fell asleep before it arrived. Henry woke me up when the delivery man came since I had cash, but I was too tired to eat. The fear that filled my stomach caused me to lose appetite for any food.

He decided to go to bed, and I laid next to him, watching him breathe. As his chest rose and fell, I couldn't imagine life without him. Even though I was the one leaving him, I still panicked knowing I would be leaving him behind on this earth.

~

Finding out I have cancer was such a hard pill to swallow. It was so exhausting and to know I have to do this every day is draining me of all my life and happiness. I left my job; I questioned my entire future. I had my first round of chemotherapy and after that I came to the conclusion that I have to do one thing which would hurt me the most.

Henry watched as I put up camp in the bathroom. Chemo gave me a run for my money, I laid on the floor of the bathroom, exhausted from vomiting every five minutes. My stomach felt as though someone threw it in the washing machine. I never felt so sick in my life. I tried everything, ginger ale, bismuth, tea, nothing stopped me from excelling liquids from every part of my body. I sipped water Henry brought me to wash down the taste of vomit. Finally, my stomach eased, and I asked Henry to warm some chicken broth. My doctor suggested I stuck to soups and soft drinks to keep the agitation of my stomach down.

I sat down with Henry at the kitchen table where the soup sat. I barely touched mine out of fear my nausea would return if I had anything in my stomach. We sat in mostly silence until I blurted out that I needed to take a halt in my life.

Quickly grabbing his attention, I said, "I think I'm going to pull my application to NYU" I said

"What...why?" he asked in a panic

"I'm not going to be able to do this." I replied, exhausted from everything.

"Why... I think you can do this. It's your lifelong dream" he said confidently as we sat at the kitchen table.

Assuring him that I wouldn't entirely give up my dreams. "I know and I'm not entirely giving it up, I just need to put it on hold until I get this under control" I replied

I assured him I wasn't going to completely abandon my goal of veterinary school. He felt relieved to know I have a goal in beating this and that I wasn't going to give up. I had him by my side, he showed me he was ready to help me take this cancer down.

I continued to sip my soup while Henry worked from home on his laptop. I watched him focus so much that I could barely get his attention. I wanted to talk to him about going back to work but he had to quickly join a conference call.

"When are you going back to work?" I asked quickly

"I'm not sure yet, I need to make sure your okay first" he replied

"I am, we need to pay the bills somehow" I assured him

"I know I'm just pulling out of saving at the moment" he said "we can talk about this later, I have to get on this call"

Henry walked away to focus on his call, and I headed back upstairs to bed. After I fell asleep, He stared at my half-full bowl of soup that I barely finished. Barely paying attention to the call, he paced the living room, pondering all that could go wrong with my diagnosis. As he watched the children playing in the street, the phone call grew louder with calls for Henry. The entire call consisted of only three people, including

Henry, was cut short after the others felt Henry's mind fueling with dark thoughts of my declining health.

~

Slumber was the only thing to keep the nausea down, but it also kept my mind busy from the constant lingering of 'cancer' in my mind. I went to my second round of chemotherapy, dreading what I knew would come following. I hated needles even as an adult and kept my eyes shut the entire time the nurses took my blood, gave me an IV, and inserted the needle into my port.

The nurse came back and told me I was ready for chemo, she handed me a ramekin of different pills. With only a small cup of water, I swallowed five different pills as I watched the nurse prepare the bags of chemotherapy. I took anti-nausea medications that just stopped me from throwing up but didn't get rid of the nauseating feeling in my stomach. I was on steroids for my fatigue that consumed my whole life.

I took a cocktail of other medications which all didn't do a lot. I sat and watched the chemo slither through the IV like a snake going to its prey. I couldn't fall asleep, so I watched as others were receiving chemo, all on such different stages of their cancer story.

"Hi" a woman sitting next to me could sense my anxiety.

She sparked a conversation trying to distract me from everything going on. She sensed my fear and tried to calm me.

"Hello, how are you- Sorry that was probably not the best thing to ask, you probably aren't great. I mean I'm not great but I'm surviving, and obviously you are... I'm sorry... I talk a lot when I'm nervous, Philomena" I said nervously.

Knowing what to say to a cancer patient was difficult. I didn't want to say the wrong thing, but I also had no idea what I was doing myself.

"Hello Philomena, Bernadette" she smiled, introducing herself in a calm, warming manner.

"Bernadette, what a pretty name" I said as I smiled back

"Thank you, I've never heard Philomena before" she replied

"Oh, it means friend of strength and courage" I
said

"How fitting" she smiled, and we continued to talk
about each other's stories.

She explained her story and it mirrored my
mother's. She had been fighting lung cancer for five
years. She offered advice and an invitation for
conversation.

Assuring me I would be okay, she told me about
her first time in chemo. She also shared her tips for
dealing with all of the symptoms that came along with
chemo drugs. Meeting someone who was there for five
years is refreshing but nerve-wracking. I can't imagine
doing this for so long but knowing I can talk to someone
is very helpful.

I walked home even though the doctors never
wanted me to, and I stopped at a coffee shop, I wanted to
get some kind of food in my system before the nausea
hit. I knew it would come up anyway, but I'll take the
short reprieve.

My doctor urged me to gain weight and increase
my calorie intake as much as possible. I couldn't keep

any kind of food down so every time I had a doctor's appointment, it was the same conversation of eating more, watching my calories, and all of the same things that I hear but can't control.

~

As I was in the coffee shop, I was reading the newspaper, I saw a zoo was up for sale and my mind started to turn. I remembered being a child, helping my grandparents with their animals.

Obviously, a zoo is a lot different, but I felt like I needed a legacy. I was so enthralled in this book that I didn't even hear the barista calling my name for my coffee. I realized my cancer will probably kill my dream of being a vet, so I decided to bring the animal career to me. I had nothing to do while being home and I feel having animals around would be therapeutic.

I decided I was going to just buy a zoo. I took the newspaper home and left it on the kitchen table. Henry didn't notice it, being so invested in my day at chemo. He couldn't come because of work so he had so many follow up questions. Every chemo appointment was the same as before, so he got the same answers. Although, he was optimistic that I wasn't sick yet. He cooked plain, grilled chicken for me, and I managed to scarf it down before I started to vomit again.

We talked about Bernadette's story. I told him how she had 5 years of experience under her belt, and she helped me through the anxiety. She was 57 years old and felt full of life. She gave me hope that I would be able to get through this. Henry was in such a happy mood knowing that I had advice from someone like Bernadette and I was also able to eat. He had no experience with sick people so he prayed I found people who were in my same grime situation who could help me through it all.

As he was cleaning up from dinner, I grabbed the newspaper from the table before he had a chance to throw it away. I laid down on the couch and reread the ad in the paper.

"Oh, so I grabbed coffee at the bodega across from the hospital today" I said leading him into a conversation about the zoo

"That's good you had that" he continued to clean up. Finishing up he sat with me on the couch.

"Yea and I was reading to the news, and I saw an article about a zoo being for sale" I replied

"What? Are you going to buy a zoo?" he laughed

"I mean..." I said, trying to get him onto my side. Convincing him that buying a zoo is not as crazy as he thinks.

"Philomena, where the hell would we find time to handle a zoo, I have a zoo of my own wrangling a bunch of middle schoolers" he argued, in a laughing tone as he really didn't believe me.

"I would take care of it" I replied seriously

"Sweetie, you stay in bed all day, or you are in the bathroom vomiting. Where are you going to find the strength to do all of that?" He replied

"I think it would help me" I assured him

He ended the conversation with the fact that we didn't have the money. Despite what he thought, I knew I had money left behind from my mother. She wasn't rich but she wanted to make sure I was taken care of after her death. I went on with my day laying in bed, puking as I always do.

But I was also doing research on buying a zoo. It was a failing private zoo, at 200 acres, that was being sold at a very low price. A lot of the animals were the grunts of the litter, the enclosures were rusted and bent out of shape, the whole zoo was falling apart.

I knew we could technically afford it in the short run, but it would be hard for the long run, especially with my cancer. So, I did what any sensible person would do, I sent a check!'

Chapter 8

I went over to my husband's school to tell him I just bought a zoo. Knowing he wouldn't be very happy, I talked with Vera for a little bit. The bell rang and Vera stopped me before I went in.

"Phil... How are you?" she asked me

"I'm doing okay, just really tired and queasy but nothing I can't handle" I replied

"Good!" she smiled

I walked to Henry's office and shut the door behind me. Knowing I wouldn't get an easy conversation out of him.

I stood at his desk, waiting for him to start the conversation. He was so infuriated that he refused to talk. I knew he was about to blow his top from looking at our bank statement.

"Henry... How are you?" I asked him.

"Can you explain the large amount of money that was taken out of our account via check for 'Brooklyn Zoo'" he asked me in an angry tone.

"Huh weird, maybe someone got a hold of our checkbook" I replied

"Philomena, what the hell?!" He yelled, throwing his head into his hands.

"Henry, I need this" I replied

"What are you going to do, how are you going to take care of all of these animals? You can barely take care of yourself! Also, where did this money come from because I know I don't make that much money!" he continued to yell.

I cut him off to explain. "I can take care of myself, you're never home to see" I said "The money comes from my mom, you don't need to worry about that, the money had nothing to do with you"

I continued to defend my actions and assure him I would be fine. He wasn't having it and continued to argue with me.

"Philomena you are sick, you cannot just go buy a zoo and take care of yourself, the animals, and the house." He argued

I assured him "No, I can handle this trust me, I will have help"

"Go home because I am very frustrated, and I can't deal with this right now" he said as he swooshed me out of his office.

He was fuming, throwing his pen across the room. While I didn't want to make him angrier, I pushed on. We continued to bicker until I finally lost it, I screamed "Of course you can't, you can never deal with anything!" He stopped, seeing my hair in the palm of my hand made him hesitate before continuing with his argument.

"Not the time Philomena!" he yelled, noticing I just created a small bald spot on the side of my head

I was so frustrated; I pulled a chunk of hair out of my scalp. It gave way so easily and I saw the effects of my chemo taking a toll on my hair now.

"There's never a time when you're too focused on work and never on me!" I yelled as I stormed out of his office.

Vera asked what was wrong. She didn't care, rather she was invested in the drama. Not much went on with work so she always enjoyed a little drama in her day.

"No! You're working for a narcissist!" I yelled at her while I rushed out to make my dramatic exit.

"Should've gone to college?" She said to herself as she continued to sneak her snacks from her locked drawer.

~

I went home, threw up in the bathroom, then I went over to Brooklyn to see this zoo I bought on a limb. It was beautiful but ominous. The greens were overgrown, animals were malnourished. I knew I had a lot to do.

Seeing this daunting task was stressful, knowing my life was turned upside down. I thought maybe Henry was right, I was in over my head, but I wanted to prove him wrong, and I was going to get this zoo up and running again. I was going to fill Brooklyn with joy again that they lost with this zoo. It seemed abandoned and no one had given a thought to it in a while. How could you just leave these animals here to die? Just starve them to death? I read the zoo went into foreclosure and declared bankruptcy, but the animals were left here, no one came back for them after closing, it seemed like such a crime.

An older gentleman came out of the main office of the zoo "Good afternoon, Philomena Williams," I introduced myself.

He was the janitor who stayed to make sure the bare minimum was being taken care of at the zoo. I could tell he didn't care and was relieved I took the burden off of his hands.

"You're the one who bought this hell hole?" he said as he organized the paperwork for me.

I looked around "I wouldn't call it that but yes" I replied

"Well good luck, there's the keys. Everything you need is in the main building at the center." He said, walking away in the sense that I lifted a weight off his shoulders.

"Well, is there anything I need to know?" I asked before he left.

"Nope, it's a shitshow, so start from scratch" he yelled.

"Got it…" I said to myself as the man left "My husbands going to kill me"

"Oh my!" I yelled as a lion roared in my ear

"Well, you are just a gorgeous little kitty... You need food" I said as I pet him through the bars.

I searched the entire zoo to see if there was any food in sight, I could only find a little, none to feed the entire zoo. I left and went to the store and chewed another large amount of money for the animals and decided to sleep at the zoo that night, knowing my husband did not want to see me. Nor did I want to talk to him. It was a cold, uncomfortable night. I slept in the old chair which was sitting in the corner of the room. As quiet as it was, I still listened to all of the animals. Some were asleep, some wide-awake scrounging for food. The entire zoo was extremely neglected, I had a lot of work to do.

I woke up to a bunch of phone calls from my husband asking where I was, I told him I was fine without telling him where I was. I still was not ready to talk to him and I knew all he would do was yell if I went home. I just did not want to deal with the constant bickering and the mindset of being dumb and not able to handle myself. I went home hoping my husband went to work and I could go home and rest in my bed while figuring out what I got myself into.

~

I thought maybe I could find people to work for me but then I realized I had to pay them. But then I figured out I could use high school students who need service hours to graduate. Yet, if I did that, I would need to talk to my husband. I knew Henry had connections with the high schools in his district.

This was difficult because I needed help, but my husband would never give me that win. I think students would eat this up though, being able to do service hours at a zoo, being able to play with animals, and be outdoors, in the fresh air. That's better than sitting in a soup kitchen or a homeless shelter. Granted, they probably need volunteers more, but I definitely need help, so I think it'll be fine, there's about ten thousand students so there's enough volunteering to go around!

Peering into his office door to see if he's cooled down. "Henry..." I said

"Philomena…" he said in a low, angry tone.

"I need your help" I asked

"Oh really?" He replied

I knew he was still very angry at me, but I wanted to still try and get him on my side. I reluctantly asked him to talk to the local high school principal, I knew I would be able to get a lot of students to help. He hesitantly agreed but had one condition…that I would come home that night. I gladly agreed as I missed my bed and the warmth of the heating.

~

I went home and made dinner. I mindlessly cooked pasta and didn't really pay attention to sanitation. I played with my hair as I was mixing everything together. This turned into spaghetti with a side of my hair that just came out in clumps without me noticing.

"You know I love you right?" He said as I made my own dish.

"Yeah, what's wrong?" I asked

Pulling a piece of my hair out of his pasta, He asked, "There's a new type of pasta now?"

I walked over, "What is that?" I asked

"Your hair" he laughed

I began to panic and ran to the bathroom to look at the mirror, I took a brush to my hair and watched as more hair came out in the brush. Each time I brushed; more hair came out. I sat, looking in the mirror, and examining my hair. I began to notice how thin and brittle my hair had become. Peering at the sink, I saw how much of my hair had fallen out.

Henry joined me in the bathroom and assured me all would be okay. He said it was all a normal thing that we knew would happen, but I couldn't help but feel embarrassed and depressed.

We walked back downstairs, and he had me sit down with him at the table, trying to have a normal meal. I didn't even want to eat at this point. I don't think Henry wanted to eat but he didn't want to upset me.

I panicked as this all became even more real. "Not a big deal?! That's my hair! I have a bald spot, Henry!"

I wasn't prepared to lose my hair, so my anxiety heightened. I knew it was going to happen, but I didn't realize it would happen so soon. I hadn't bought a wig or any head scarves. I also didn't want to shave my head, nor did I want to keep my hair with chunks missing. I just didn't want to lose my hair…

Henry continuously comforted me as hair quickly fell out in clumps, in the kitchen, the bathroom, and in the shower; I found hair in my car, and my purse, my poor husband had hair in his food. I never thought it would be so difficult to find my long blonde hair everywhere I went. My life was changing so much. In such insignificant ways.

I woke up the next day feeling like I was thrown around on a rollercoaster. I spent the morning laying on the bathroom floor, and I mustered the energy to make it to the kitchen to make lunch, which did not last long in my stomach. I knew I needed to eat but my throat was so burnt from the constant vomit coming up. I did learn that plain chicken broth without salt stays down the most, so I continued to just sip it alone.

So far, I had lost 6 pounds and was officially under 100 pounds. I was always a tiny person, but I didn't expect to be so frail. My clothes were baggy, I couldn't put my shoes on without help.

I decided to take a nap which turned into a 14-hour sleep. When Henry got home, he didn't wake me up and I didn't even realize when he got home. I was worried he was missing work, but he expressed concern for my declining health. I was in such a deep sleep; he couldn't wake me up which worried him enough to stay home from work.

He knew I had chemo later that day but pressured me to cancel it. During the night I woke up to throw up and couldn't make it to the toilet. Henry managed to clean everything up but was worried I wasn't ready for another round of chemotherapy.

As he helped me change out of my vomit-ridden clothes, he asked me to skip chemo. I refused knowing that would just delay the inevitable. I wanted to get through chemo so badly and I didn't care if it would make me so sick I couldn't function.

I continued to throw up, mid chemo and they decided to prescribe me new anti-nausea medication. I wasn't sure the actual point of the medication, but it stopped me from throwing up yet didn't get rid of the nauseating feeling in the pit of my stomach. I also tried anti-nausea lollipops which also did not work. I learned to deal with the pain because I understood it wasn't going away. My doctors pushed different medications that didn't help, and it was exhausting to keep trying different ones.

Chapter 9

Getting up to get ready for the day became more and more difficult as each day went by. I got up, brushed my teeth, threw up, and swished with mouthwash to try and get rid of the taste of vomit. Then I threw a head wrap on and started my day. Typically, I stayed home, went to the zoo, or went to visit Henry at work. On this particular day, I decided to visit Henry at work and bring him some lunch as a peace offering since I had bought an entire zoo without his input.

I was sitting in the main office when Vera came inside from a smoke break. My mind was immediately taken back to the days of my mother always lighting one up as I smelled her cigarettes fill the room. I watched as she sprayed perfume all over herself to mask the smell of tobacco.

"Did I ever tell you about my mom?" I asked her. My mom was the reason I never touched a cigarette. Despite that, I guess it didn't matter since cancer got me anyway.

"Nope" she chuckled

"She died of lung disease from smoking cigarettes" I replied

She quickly changed the conversation knowing she was probably down the same exact path.

"Anyway... I heard you bought a zoo??" she said

"I bought a zoo" I replied with blind confidence

I told her how I was ditching my vet school dreams for now and taking a different direction for my now short life. She laughed at me, calling me crazy. Maybe I was but she would be biting her words once I get this zoo off the ground.

She quickly noticed my somber demeanor, realizing I wasn't my usual cheerful self. Concern crept into her usually cold tone as she sensed something was wrong. For once in our short relationship, she seemed concerned for me, with how sick I was. Reluctant to delve into the heaviness of my terminal diagnosis, I shut her down and asked her to get my husband.

Everyone was so focused on me that no one checked up on Henry. He's always had a strong will but there's only so far, a person can be pushed before their breaking point. I needed to make sure Henry wouldn't hit his breaking point because I needed him to stay strong when I couldn't. She assured me he was doing well. I believe he was distracting himself with work. Trying to keep busy so he couldn't think of the world around him.

~

Vera told me Henry was in a meeting and I ended up leaving so I didn't need to sit in the main office talking to her. I left for the zoo, trying to keep my mind off of my cancer. I took the subway over, and once I got there, I watched all the animals scrounging for food. I grabbed the bucket of a mixture of nuts and fruits and headed to the enclosures.

I watched the monkeys climbing the trees as my voice grew softer, tinged with a mixture of sadness and acceptance.

"You know, little friend, there's a strange comfort in sitting here with you, knowing that life goes on even as mine slips away. It's as if your playful antics remind me the world keeps spinning, even when my own journey is nearing its end."

As I watched the babies swing from branch to branch, I couldn't help but marvel at the resilience of life. In their world, there was no room for sorrow or regret, just the instinct to survive and thrive. Perhaps that was a lesson I could take with me as I faced what lay ahead.

I knew I might not have had much time left, but in moments like those, I found solace in the simple joys of existence. The warmth of the sun on my skin, the sound of laughter in the distance, and the gentle companionship of creatures like you. The zoo helped me see all of these things in the world.

I got a sharp pain in my gut as I was feeding all of these animals. I tried to ignore it but after a while, it continued to get worse, and I decided to head home. I hid my pain from Henry because I didn't want to worry him any more than what he was already. Eventually, he figured something was up, but I refused to tell him. I never liked worrying people if I could handle it myself. I also didn't want to face the possible reality of the fact that it could be my cancer spreading. If my cancer was spreading, I knew my chances of beating this would continue to slim.

My heart felt heavy as my mind continued to swirl with thoughts of a terminal diagnosis. Henry continuously asked me if I was okay and I brushed him off, trying to not worry him, despite seeing the pain I was in. I convinced him to go to bed while I stayed up trying to find a remedy to my pain.

I couldn't get a minute of sleep in as the pain continued to get worse. I decided to wake my husband up after I noticed blood in my pee. My period wasn't due, and I knew I wasn't pregnant so all that could race through my mind was my cancer had spread.

We had walked to the hospital and the emergency room was filled with people coming from all different walks of life. I felt so terrified as Henry continued to assure me everything would be fine. Every time I visited the hospital, the employees always were so professional, with not an ounce of fear or anxiety in their voices. They knew how to make people seem as though nothing was wrong, and we were overreacting in a sense.

Henry grew frustrated with me and my conversations of dread so I decided to stop talking knowing he would snap at me pretty soon. We sat in silence waiting and watching all of the other people in the same room with completely different lives. A New York emergency room will always be the most insane place, especially amidst the dead of the night.

After an hour of waiting, we were called back. I explained how I was in agonizing pain and my urine was filled with blood. She seemed to act as though nothing was a major concern until Henry mentioned my cancer. The doctor then got a urine sample which was more like a blood sample.

Henry continued to try and calm me as I argued about how calm the doctor had seemed. He explained that she's been doing this all her life and she's probably seen this before. He gently stroked my arm, then held my hand tightly. I pulled away; I was so frustrated that he could see the reality of the situation.

"I can't Henry, how am I supposed to relax, please explain to me, I'd love to know!"

I continued to argue with Henry as he tried to reason with me. I couldn't stop thinking about how my cancer had most likely spread. No one would outright tell me but I'm sure they were all thinking the same. I knew at this point my cancer was in my breast and lymph nodes. I was looking at a late stage III and I knew if my cancer had spread then I would progress to a stage VI which would be terminal.

I had extensive scans and endless tests to tell me the inevitable. The doctors finally came in and showed my scans without explaining them in layman's terms.

Another doctor came into the room and briefly paused before asking the question I dreaded the most. "Has your doctor ever explained the causes or probability of your cancer spreading?"

"No…not entirely" my husband replied as I stared blankly at him.

"Okay, well we did find mets in your stomach, liver, and kidneys. Ultimately, putting you through surgery at this point would do more harm than good. We need to look at each situation and see the bad outweighing the good"

"Okay… so I'm a dead man walking…how long… am I looking at" I interjected, barely able to get my words out. My heart began to race and my anxiety soared.

"No, not necessarily. Your primary oncologist will most likely increase your chemo regimen and will likely put you on radiotherapy as well. There are also numerous clinical trials you can possibly be a good candidate for." he said optimistically

I began to grab my things. "Okay well thank you, we should be heading home" I said

I hadn't fully processed what he had said, and I just wanted to go home like the trip never even happened.

"Philomena, relax, I have more questions" Henry told me

"We will put you on a high dose of pain medication to help with the pain" the doctor explained

"Great, so I'll be in less pain physically, more pain emotionally, thank you so much!" I laughed grimly

"Philomena!" Henry yelled.

I ignored both of them, I quickly got changed and ran home, completely distraught. All Henry wanted to do was talk about it but all I wanted to do was ignore it.

"Can we please talk?" Henry asked as I stormed upstairs.

I yelled no and slammed my door, locking it from behind. He sat at the door, talking through the crease. He continued to assure me everything would be okay, and I could fight this.

I continued to ignore him, yelling "Goodnight!" each time he would bring up a new conversation. I sat in a quiet corner of my room, gazing out the window at the birds, my thoughts drifting to the resilience of the natural world.

It's funny how life can mirror the cycles of nature, isn't it? We're all just animals navigating our way through the wilderness of existence, facing trials and tribulations along the way. And like the creatures of the forest, sometimes we're confronted with obstacles that seem insurmountable.

I watched a bird perched on a nearby branch, its wings spread wide as it took flight. But even in the face of adversity, there's a remarkable resilience that emerges. Look at the way the bird soars through the sky, despite the storms it may encounter. It's a reminder that strength isn't just about physical prowess, but the unwavering determination to keep moving forward, no matter the odds.

In a way, I'm like that bird, navigating through the storms of life with grace and courage. Yes, the path ahead may be fraught with uncertainty, but I refuse to be defined by fear or despair. I'll spread my wings and fly, embracing each moment as a precious gift, knowing that even in the darkest of times, there's beauty to be found in the simplest of joy.

Chapter 10

The job of revamping the zoo was a daunting one that I knew I couldn't do alone. I employed the job of my niece to help me. Daisy was 18 and from my husband's side. His older sister had a child who was currently going to school for Piano in New York.

She was a sweet, vivacious girl who was more than willing to help anyone in need. I knew she was perfect to get to help me. We shared a common love of animals, and she needed things to put on her resume, so it was a win-win.

Without Henry's knowledge, I headed up to Lincoln Center to go speak with Daisy. I was walking around campus, and I could tell why she spent so much money on tuition and housing. The extravagance of the campus made me feel a sense of sadness that I made never experience this in my own way with veterinary school.

I met her in an old practice room where she was preparing for an exam. Exams were very different than when I was in college, I guess because I wasn't in a performing arts school. As much as I wanted to say it looked easier, I knew I could never do what she was doing. I listened to her practicing, and it was just so beautiful, I forgot why I was even there.

"Hey Mena, what are your thoughts?" she said as she finished an elegant Italian piece.

"It's so beautiful, I am…so impressed!" I replied

"Aw! Thank you, I've been trying to make it flow more but it's just not working with me," she said "Anyway, what's up? I saw your text but was honestly kind of confused"

"Oh, it flows fine, trust me! But today… so I'm sure you know about my cancer?" I asked in a way that was so casual and I didn't need to cry yet again.

"Oh my god, yes, my dad told me about it, I'm so sorry!! How are you doing? Do you need any help at home or anything?" she replied

"Oh no I'm okay, I have been going through chemo and staying on top of my doctors' notes so I'm on the right track, thank you for asking!" I assured her.

"So, what brings you to Lincoln Center?" She asked as she quietly played

"Well, I bought a zoo!" I replied

"What?" she laughed

"Yes! And I was really hoping I could get your help. If not, trust me I get it, you are busy with school and have your own life" I replied

"No, no! I actually would love to! That sounds so exciting! Where? What? When? Why?" she said eccentrically

"It's in Brooklyn, an old zoo that needs a lot of work. I realized after my cancer diagnosis I couldn't go to school full time, but I can't just sit home sulking, so I bought it!" I explained

"Oh my god, I love it! Count me in!" she smiled

We walked to her dorm and set out a plan for what to do with the zoo. I knew I wanted to bring it back to what it was and open it back to the public. I just needed to get Daisy up to speed.

She lived on the 12th floor of her dorm, with a gorgeous view of the Manhattan skyline.

"What's your cost of living here?" I asked

"About 22k a year," she said ever so casually

"Shit, that's crazy, just for housing?!" I exclaimed.

Pulling a bottle of cheap tequila from under her

"Yes, I pay almost 90k a year in total" she replied,

"Wow… well maybe the zoo could help that, or not but if anything, it'll be something!" I said as she offered me a tequila and orange juice.

"So, what's your plan??" She asked me

"Honestly, I have no idea!" I laughed, peering out at the Manhattan skyline from her dorm window.

"Ok cool, so we're starting from the beginning" she said

"Yes, we are!" I smiled, cheering with the 2 glasses of cheap tequila at three o'clock in the afternoon.

We sat in her dorm, planning the next few months to get the zoo back up and running. I pulled out the plans that were given to me by the janitor. They were all stained and ripped and hard to read so we had to improvise a lot.

We rewrote all of the paperwork to fit our needs and created a new map that didn't have any questionable stains or missing pieces. It took a lot of time and effort, but we managed to organize all of the information we needed.

~

Later that day, I headed home to talk with Henry. I showed him all of the paperwork Daisy and I constructed, and he seemed to slowly work with me and get the feel of my ideas. Thinking that maybe I could pull this off even with cancer.

Henry hadn't seen Daisy in a while even though they lived so close by. Henry wasn't close with his sister, so he never really was involved with Daisy's life. I didn't want to stir the pot between Henry and his sister, so I tried to not bring up a lot about it.

"So, how's Daisy?" Henry asked.

"She's good, let me just tell you! She is amazing at the piano!" I said happily

"I know, I remember listening to her when she was a kid, I don't know where she got it because no one in my family has any musical ability"

"That's what I thought too!"

We dropped the topic of his sister's family quite quickly and moved on to the zoo template. I showed him a brief outline of what our plans were. We had a lion enclosure, a monkey tree playground, and an indoor area for insects and amphibians. An outdoor theatre that was attached to an education center. A pond with ducks, turtles, and an array of nature that you find in any water. We added an aquatics department as well. We have a sea lion habitat and aquatic birds, and we really wanted to get a dolphin exhibit as well.

We wanted to create a children's place as well to attract more families. Having a small playground or an interactive space for children would be so beneficial for parents and kids alike. As well as a playground, we decided to implement a weekly learning session at the education center for the children to interact with different animals. It took time but we came up with a rough draft of a template as well as a picture of all that we had envisioned.

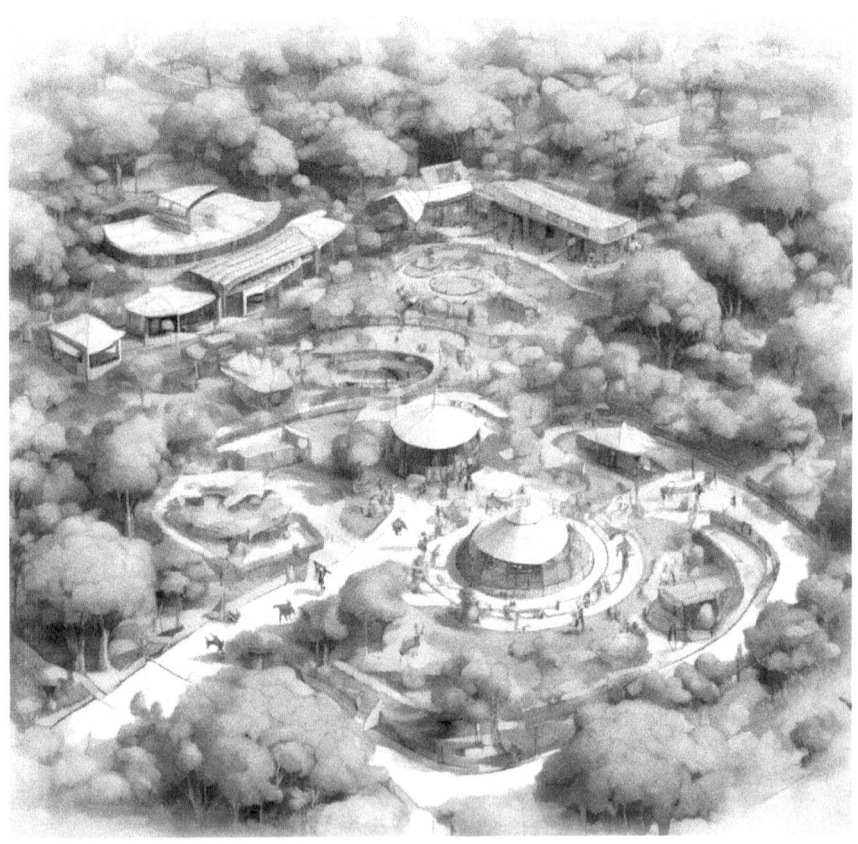

With all of these plans, chemo made it difficult to actually set them into play. I was always so weak, so I didn't have the strength to do heavy labor. A lot of the physical stuff had to be done by Daisy while I handled the paperwork like budgets and finding out where to get animals for the zoo. A lot of the animals came with the zoo, but some did not like the sea lions or dolphins we had plans for.

I never thought about how people would buy animals to open a zoo, so I spent most of my days on a computer researching where to buy animals from that wasn't the black market or China. It was a nice distraction from being constantly sick. I was able to change my focus and bring myself to a more confident environment. I believe God gave me this zoo for a reason, for me to help these animals and for the animals to help me get through cancer.

~

Christmas was quickly approaching, and the winter was treating everyone as harshly as always. The piercing wind and icy temperatures were taking a toll on my frail body. It was difficult to leave the house and be outside at the zoo. Fortunately, I had Daisy do a lot of the outdoor work, while I stayed inside to do paperwork.

"My goodness, it is cold!" Daisy said after coming inside from working.

"I know when I came inside, I couldn't feel my fingers!" I replied

"Yea I mean the polar bears are in heaven though" she laughed

"Awe, that's adorable, I'll have to head over there." I said, "Did you hear it's supposed to snow on Christmas Eve?"

"Really? That's exciting!" she replied

"Yeah, it'll be nice to have my last Christmas be a white Christmas," I said

"Don't say that!" She argued

"Okay, okay… possibly my last" I said

She assured me "No… you will have more!"

I always loved Christmas time and to be in New York for this year makes this time even more magical. It was unfathomable to imagine that this would be my first Christmas and possibly my last here in the city.

Henry and I sat at home for Christmas because I was too sick to travel home to Illinois. So many people asked me what I wanted for Christmas, but I couldn't think of anything but a new body which wasn't riddled with tumors. My dad came to the city to celebrate Christmas as well as to take the load off of Henry. It was a very low-key Christmas, we went to church, the three of us, and then Henry and my dad cooked dinner together while I slept.

When New years eve rolled around, I couldn't stay awake for the ball drop and slept into the new year. Henry watched the ball drop on TV while in bed with me. My dad had to head back to Illinois because of work but he had thoughts about coming back full time to help me and Henry. While it was a new year, it was the same, old chemo, doctors, and appointments.

Chapter 11

In a dimly lit hospital room, the flickering fluorescent lights cast eerie shadows across my face as I lay in the bed. The IV dripped steadily, delivering a potent cocktail of chemotherapy drugs, and I braced myself for the onslaught of side effects that inevitably followed.

Nausea crept in like a relentless tide, threatening to consume me whole. Every muscle ached, and every joint felt weighed down by an invisible burden as if the very ounce of strength I had was being slowly drained away.

But it wasn't just the physical toll that weighed heavy on my shoulders. It was the knowledge that this treatment, while necessary, came with a price that few could fully comprehend. The loss of my hair, once a symbol of my youth, served as an evident reminder of the battle raging within my body. The fatigue, so profound even the simplest tasks felt like insurmountable obstacles wore down my happiness like a relentless hammer pounding against a hard stone. What was the point of it all if I was only delaying the inevitable? Yet, amidst the darkness, there were flickers of hope. The whispered words of encouragement from loved ones, the gentle touch of a nurse's hand offering comfort in the midst of chaos. And above all, there was my unwavering determination to fight, to cling to life with every ounce of strength I possessed. In the depths of despair, there was a glimmer of light, a slim possibility of better days ahead.

~

My dad decided to move to NY with us the minute I was diagnosed with cancer. He had a bit of experience from my mom, I think I gave him a little PTSD from my diagnosis. I loved having him here, but it was a little bigot suffocating so he ultimately rented his own apartment nearby. He was available but not on top of us.

Despite my cancer diagnosis, I still wanted to live my life and at least, try to go on with my normal self.

My dad was a college professor who taught history and mom was a high school teacher. Even though he didn't know much about medical terms or hospital lingo, he was still great to have for moral support.

My name came from my dad, his parents were Greek immigrants and came through Ellis Island. My grandmother's name is Philomena, which means, friend of strength. My grandmother lived her name through living in NY, then moving to Illinois without knowing a lick of English. I was always honored to be named after her and now I had to find my own strength in my different battle of cancer. Deep down, I wanted to find the strength she had, as different as it may have been.

After chemo, my dad and I went to a small café to get a snack before the nausea set in. It was a nice little outing where we both ignored my cancer and had a father-daughter lunch. A spring day in Central Park Cafe was a delightful experience. As we sat at a cozy table on the patio, the gentle warmth of the sun filtered through the budding leaves of surrounding trees. The air was fresh, filled with the scents of blooming flowers and the distant sound of children playing and birds chirping. The cafe buzzed with a pleasant hum of conversations, accompanied by the clinking of cups and the aroma of freshly brewed coffee. Tulips and daffodils added splashes of color to the lush green landscape, creating a vibrant and inviting atmosphere perfect for enjoying a peaceful moment in nature's embrace.

I was terrified to eat so I ordered a small salad with a black coffee, and my dad had a chicken club. It was a great salad, fresh herbs and greens. I could tell my dad loved his club from his lack of talking and abundance of chews I heard. I slowly sipped my coffee and ate only half of my salad before subtly bolting to the bathroom to throw up in the bathroom. Thankfully it was a private bathroom and not many people were there. So, I found there can of air freshener and drowned the bathroom in it so no one could tell I committed. Except my dad could tell since my face was red and eyes were watery. He didn't say a word about it knowing it was basically a normal occurrence at this point. After awhile it became a silent assumption that when I got sick, I was fine unless I asked for someone's help. I hated to be a burden to people, so I tried to keep my problems to myself.

~

After enduring another grueling session of chemotherapy and a small lunch with my dad, I finally returned home, feeling utterly drained both physically and emotionally. Collapsing onto my bed, I sank into the familiar warmth of soft blankets and plush pillows, seeking refuge from the relentless pain within me. Every movement sent waves of exhaustion coursing through my weary body, and I found myself longing for nothing more than the simple comfort of stillness.

As I lay there in the quiet solitude of my room, I let out a heavy sigh, feeling the weight of the world pressing down on my shoulders. At that moment, all I could do was surrender to the overwhelming fatigue and allow myself the luxury of rest, knowing tomorrow would bring with it a new day and the strength to face whatever challenges lay ahead.

Henry, home after a long day at work, walked into my dark room, he asked how my chemo session went.

"It was tough. I'm really feeling drained and nauseous." I responded from under the covers.

"I'm sorry, love. Is there anything I can do to help?"

He walked over to my side, gently pulling the sheets from my head. The small ounce of light that peered in from behind the curtains caused my head to throb.

"Just having you here with me means the world. But maybe you could grab me some ginger tea? It usually helps settle my stomach."

"Of course, I'll go make some right now. And don't worry about anything else today. Just focus on resting and taking care of yourself. Daisy is taking care of everything with the zoo"

I responded with tears in my eyes "Thank you, honey. I don't know what I'd do without you by my side through all of this."

"We're in this together, remember? I'll always be here for you, no matter what." he went downstairs and made my tea.

I only drank half as my stomach was turning, my lips were so chapped it burned to sip anything but water. We wished each other goodnight, and an 'I love you' before he had a peaceful night's sleep, and I had a night of bouncing between the bathroom and bedroom.

~

The next day, I woke up feeling slightly better after yesterday's grueling chemo session. Though still fatigued and achy, the oppressive weight that seemed to suffocate me had lifted ever so slightly, allowing me to breathe a little easier. With each passing hour, I found myself slowly regaining a sense of normalcy, savoring the small victories like being able to eat a few bites of toast without feeling nauseous. As the sun filtered through the curtains, casting a warm glow across the room, I couldn't help but feel a renewed sense of hope stirring within me. That day may still have been challenging, but for then, I cherished that fleeting reprieve and held onto the promise of brighter days ahead.

As I walked towards the zoo on a glorious spring day, the warmth of the sun enveloped me like a comforting embrace, chasing away the lingering chill of winter. The streets were alive with the hustle and bustle of people, their faces alight with smiles as they reveled in the beauty of the season. Children skipped alongside their parents, their laughter echoing through the air like music to my ears. With each step, I felt a sense of anticipation building within me, eager to immerse myself in the wonders that awaited me at the zoo. It was a day filled with promise and possibility, I was excited to get back to the zoo and prepare for the summer, school field trips, family vacations, and so much more.

I watched Daisy come running over, excited as ever to see me. "Can you believe the opening day is just a few weeks away?!" she excitedly said

Trying to contain her excitement, I said, "I know, but there's still so much to do before then."

"Tell me about it. We've got to finalize the exhibits, hire more staff, and make sure everything is in tip-top shape!"

We sat in the office, contemplating all that we needed to do. We planned an opening day as well as planning the next few weeks. Working my chemo schedule and doctors' appointments into it.

"And don't forget about promoting the grand opening! We want to make sure the whole city knows about our zoo." Daisy interjected.

I forgot we would even need to promote in the community. I thought it would all just come naturally but Daisy reminded me that practically everyone forgot about this zoo after closing.

"I have faith we'll pull it off. We've come this far, and we are so close to the finish line!"

"That's the spirit! Together, we'll make this zoo the pride of the city. I can't wait to see the smiles on people's faces when they walk through our gates for the first time."

The next few weeks we spent endless hours cleaning, building, and refurbishing the entire zoo. Even though I was so sick, we were able to do everything ahead of schedule. Daisy made sure to keep everything on schedule even when I was not there.

"Hello, I'm Philomena, the owner of this zoo. I have a decent understanding of otters, but I know you're the expert when it comes to their medical care. Can you share some insights on their health and well-being? I want to make sure we have a thriving community of these guys." I said as we sat down in the office.

"Nice to meet you, Philomena. Absolutely, I specialize in otter healthcare. Otters are fascinating creatures, and ensuring their good health is crucial. From dental care to dietary needs and overall wellness, I'm here to provide the best possible medical support for them." He replied

"That's reassuring to hear!"

"It's so cool to think that you specifically work with otters! They seem to have such complex needs. What are some common health issues they face that we should be looking out for?" I asked

I was intensively writing notes down, I only had the knowledge from my bachelor's, but I wanted to be able to gain more knowledge, all the things I would learn in vet school.

"Indeed, they do. Otters can be susceptible to various health issues, including dental problems, respiratory infections, and parasites. Regular check-ups and preventive measures are essential to keep them healthy and thriving in their habitat." He replied

We continued to talk about the otters as well as getting his coworkers in to help with other animals. I wanted to make sure each species had the utmost care.

After our meeting, I gave him a tour of the zoo and introduced him to Daisy. He saw all of the work we were doing for the zoo and commended us on our hard work and dedication to the animals.

"Thank you for your dedication to the otters' well-being. It's comforting to know they're in capable hands. I'll ensure we provide all the necessary support for their medical care." I responded

"You're welcome! I look forward to working with you to ensure these wonderful creatures lead long, healthy lives here at the zoo. I will also get back to you on the information for others to come help you with different animals as well!" He said as I led him out.

I had to do that for every animal, it was exhausting but I managed. Before buying the zoo, I never thought of all the upkeep and third-party people I would need to bring in to maintain the health and wellness of all animals. It was super expensive and laborious, but it all paid off in the end.

Chapter 12

Despite battling a terminal illness, after months of tireless dedication and unwavering passion, I stood at the entrance of my newly refurbished zoo, my heart swelling with pride and anticipation. My determination is undeterred by the shadow of my own mortality.

Each enclosure, meticulously designed and lovingly crafted, was a testament to my vision of creating a sanctuary where both animals and visitors could thrive in harmony. Knowing I might not witness the zoo's full potential unfold, I found purpose amidst my pain. The gates swung open on that long-awaited opening day, and a wave of excitement rippled through the crowd, eager to explore the wonders that awaited within. With a sense of fulfillment coursing through my veins, I watched as families and children embarked on a journey of discovery, their laughter and wonderment echoing through the air.

It was the beginning of a legacy built on a foundation of compassion, conservation, and boundless imagination. For me, this zoo was more than just a legacy; it was a symbol of resilience, a beacon of hope that transcended my existence, however short it might be.

As I watched all of the visitors, I heard the distant voice of my lovely husband. We stood together pondering on all I did. Sitting beside Henry, I was overwhelmed by a wave of gratitude and pride as we reflected on my accomplishments despite my terminal diagnosis. Each milestone felt like a victory, a testament to the resilience of the human spirit. I was confident in the impact I've made, the lives I've touched, and the legacy I've created in such a short time.

At that moment, surrounded by the unwavering support of my loved ones, I was filled with a sense of peace and purpose, knowing that my journey, though challenging, has been filled with moments of triumph and joy. Together Henry and I found strength in each other's embrace, cherishing the memories we've created and the love that binds us together, even in the face of adversity.

It took months of preparing, but I managed to turn a disheveled zoo into the talk of Brooklyn. I honestly didn't think I could do it with everything going on with the cancer and all. Yet somehow, I did it… I did this... Just like me and my health, I took on the task of building up this dilapidated zoo that was at risk of failing all of these animals. My body was failing me, and I am taking the task to build it back up.

People came from all over the five boroughs. I couldn't help but feel an overwhelming sense of joy and appreciation. These people came for me and my animals, my volunteers' dedication to helping me, it's just so mind-blowing that this all came together.
I began my speech to all of the eager patrons,

I honestly did not think I would make it to this point, but I feel blessed beyond words. Today marks not only the opening of a new, fresh haven for wildlife, but the celebration of life and resilience. As someone who has faced the trials of cancer, I stand before you with a heart full of gratitude and determination. This zoo is not just a testament to survival, but a symbol of hope and the indomitable spirit that resides in all of us. We have built more than enclosures and pathways here; we've created a sanctuary where the majesty of nature can foster joy, curiosity, and a deep appreciation for the preciousness of life. Each animal here, from the smallest insect to the grandest elephant, is a reminder of the diversity and resilience of life on Earth

To everyone who has supported this journey, your belief has been my strength. To my husband, thank you for your unwavering support through all of this, I know it cannot be easy dealing with me, but I'm beyond grateful to you… and your checkbook. To my volunteers, thank you, I know that you were doing this for service hours, but I feel I can say we had a lot of fun! To visitors, may you find here the same sense of wonder and courage has carried me through my darkest days. Together, let's embark on this adventure, not just to

observe, but to learn and to emerge stronger, kinder, and more connected to the natural world around us.
Thank you, and let the wild wonders begin!

"Good job Mrs. Williams!" an old student of Henry's said.

She had come before Henry became an administrator and taught high school-level chemistry. School brought her to the city to study law.

"Thanks, sweetie! How have you been?" I replied.

"Good! I miss your husband's crazy experiments. I still tell people about when he almost burnt the building down" she said

"Oh, trust me, he hasn't stopped!" I laughed

I'm not surprised in the slightest!" She laughed "I had a lot of fun, and I was wondering if maybe you had an opening position for a job. Law school is getting pretty stressful, so I need to find something to help." she asked hesitantly.

"As a matter of fact, I do, and I would love to be able to have you work with me! I know you probably assumed I need a lot more employees" I smiled.

"Thank you! Yeah, I know it is probably hard to start something from the ground up." she said happily. She told me about growing up in this zoo. How when she was a child, the zoo was thriving and so many people came from all over. It was so cool to hear a story from when the zoo was actually in working condition

"My dad used to take us here every Sunday when my mom was working day shifts at the hospital, my favorites were always the otters. They just were always so funny and adorable."

"Yes, they're so cute! I made sure to keep them when we were looking at the animals to bring in. We brought them in from Canada."

~

As I was talking to all of the visitors, I found my husband watching from afar. He was taking a stroll through the zoo to witness all that I had done.
"I'm Proud of you" he said as he put his arm around my shoulder.

"I'm proud of me too," I said, "And I'm proud of you!"

"Why do you say that? You made all of this happen." he asked, kissing my forehead.

"I know, but you stood by me, you didn't give up on my crazy ideas. I can only imagine how tough it must be for you to see me go through this." I smiled and grabbed his hand. "Let's go get some drinks next to the lion's den." I continued

"I never thought alcohol and lions would be in the same sentence." he laughed as we walked, hand in hand, to the outdoor bar.

Henry,

It takes an incredible amount of strength and love to be there for someone during such a difficult time, but let me tell you my friend, you are doing an amazing job.

Taking care of your wife means more than just being by her side physically. It means being her rock, her support system, and her source of comfort when things get tough. It's about being there to listen, to hold her hand, and to remind her that she's not alone in this battle.

Remember, it's okay to feel overwhelmed sometimes. It's a lot to handle, and you're only human, but don't forget to take care of yourself too. You need to recharge and stay strong for both of you. Lean on your support network, whether it's family, friends, or a support group. They can provide a listening ear, advice, and a shoulder to lean on.

Above all, keep the love and hope alive. Celebrate the small victories, cherish the moments of joy, and keep fighting together. Your love and care are invaluable to your wife, and they will make a difference in her journey.

Thank you, Henry

As Henry and I were sitting at the outside bar, we heard someone running down the path in our direction. We saw Daisy come into view, busting from excitement.

"We did it, we did it, we did it!!!" Daisy said as she ran over to me and Henry.

"Ahh! Yes, we did!" I yelled

"Daisy, it's great to see you!" Henry interjected, surprised to see his niece after so long.

Henry was not very close with his sister so that lack of communication stemmed from his niece, Daisy. They were able to rekindle their relationship despite his sister's absence. Even though they now lived in the same city, they had not seen each other since Daisy was 11.

"Uncle Henry, how are you?" She said as she leaned in for a hug.

"Doing good, thanks for helping my wife with her crazy ideas!" Henry laughed

"Hey! My crazy ideas are paying our bills!" I interjected

"She's not wrong" Daisy laughed

She went and ordered a drink and sat down with us, bringing us drinks as well.

"How old are you?" I asked, knowing she was just a sophomore in college.

"In New York? 19, but in Jersey, I'm 24" she said

"Oh great!" Henry laughed

"So, what are your plans for the future?" Henry asked, trying to catch up with his niece.

"Well, I'm going to graduate with a piano degree, and I'll probably stay here while playing in concerts" she replied, "Maybe Broadway if I'm lucky"

"Wow! Good for you, I'm sure your mom is so proud!" Henry smiled

"She is, she doesn't know about the zoo part though, so I'll tell her eventually," Daisy said

"Your sister doesn't know about me?" I asked Henry

"I guess not, we don't really talk" he replied

"She knows about your cancer but not the zoo" Daisy interjected

Their laugher echoed through the air, merging with the chatter of the animals. As Daisy and Henry's bond grew stronger, I felt as though the zoo itself came alive with newfound hope and vitality. I had hoped it could bring more families and friends together just as it did with Henry and his niece.

For me, the building of this reunion, every moment was both a triumph and a reminder of my terminal label. Despite the joy I brought to others, the shadow of my illness loomed large, casting a dark curtain over my accomplishments. The knowledge that I might never witness the zoo's full potential weighed heavily on my heart, a poignant reminder of life's most precious moments. Yet, in the face of this uncertainty, my unwavering faith in Daisy and her ability to carry on my legacy was a beacon of hope, illuminating the path forward even in the darkest of time.

Chapter 13

Juggling cancer and a zoo isn't the easiest but it was
great to have people in my circle. When I had chemo,
Henry stayed by my side, Daisy was at the zoo, and Vera
helped Henry with being able to do work from home or
the hospital. I sat in the bedroom waiting for Henry to
leave. Once he left, I was planning on going back to
sleep, but he was taking his sweet time while changing.

"I can't stand this stupid chemo!" I yelled from
across the room.

Henry was quickly changing for work as he was
running late from helping me with my medications. The
medications were scattered across the kitchen counter so

Henry could organize all of my morning medications. I grabbed his hand and swiped the medications all over the floor. Luckily, each bottle had an individual description of the pill so Henry had to inspect every single pill. As he was cleaning it all up, I continued to argue with him about taking my medications that only caused me more pain and suffering.

He was crawling all over the floor to clean up my medications, while I hid from him refusing to take a single one. "Well, it's helping you!" he replied.

"Is it though?" I said.

"Yes! Stop acting like you are on death's doorstep." he laughed

I helped him grab all of his things. Making sure he remembered the lunch that I made him the night before. I was not laughing at his lightness of the entire situation.

"But I am Henry, just face it. I am dying." I said.

He quickly changed the subject to hear my plans for the day.

"See I told you." I said without answering his question.

"What?!"

"That I am dying, and you don't want to admit it."

He began to grow frustrated with me as I refused to let go of his lack of empathy. "I'm not having this conversation, I'm late for work."

Henry reluctantly grabbed his bags, keys, and coat, then left for work without having a single conversation with me about my death. He was already late for work and I knew I lost my time to sit in bed waiting to go to my own job.

~

I left for the zoo at 8 am sharp to open the doors by ten. That hour before was so loud with birds screeching, alpacas spitting, as well as lions roaring while I mounted the food in the bin.

Within the zoo, there existed a unique harmony between the silence and the vibrant noise of animal life. Before the bustling tones of visitors, the air was alive with the lively chatter of various animals, each contributed their own distinct voice to the symphony of sounds. From the gentle rustle of leaves in the monkey enclosure to the melodic calls of tropical birds in the aviary, the atmosphere is teeming with life. In this sanctuary of serenity, one finds a rare blend of solitude and liveliness, a testament to the peaceful coexistence between humans and the magnificent creatures that call the zoo home.

The hour spent alone with nothing, but the animals was remarkably quiet. It granted me a sense of solitude in the company of nature's creatures. I didn't need therapy; I confided my troubles to the monkeys and seeking solace amidst the tigers. Although met with silence, the act of unburdening myself provided a sense of ease. I found no necessity for well-intentioned, but ultimately hollow assurances from family members regarding my prognosis. Acknowledging the reality of my terminal illness, I sought comfort in the simple act of being present for the animals, providing them with care and sustenance.

As the clock struck ten the gates opened to admit a steady stream of visitors. I observed with fondness the diverse array of individuals, from elderly couples leisurely observing the otters, to energetic toddlers eager to explore every exhibit, their stuffed companions in tow. Amidst the hustle and bustle, I reveled in the opportunity to share the wonders of the zoo with others.

On this particular day, I had a 4th grade class coming for a field trip. They were traveling from Queens which, with traffic, was about an hour's drive. I knew having 40 fourth graders on a bus for an hour was anyone's nightmare. I wanted to make sure everything was as smooth as possible for the teachers and chaperones.

"Okay, is everything ready?" I asked Daisy in a panic.

"Yes, maps are set out for each group, groups are set out for chaperones to have six students each. Also, lunch will be ready at 12:30 in the parks. Groups will all be joined together for lunch."

She assured me everything was set up and organized for this class trip.

"Perfect, thank you so so much!" I hugged her.

"That's my job!" she smiled.

"By the way, are you doing, okay?" she asked me even though I could not bear to answer.

"I'm fine, don't ask again." I replied

"Noted." she said, dropping the conversation quickly.

I wasn't feeling great, but I didn't want to be reminded of it, so I just wanted to keep my looming tribulations of cancer out of the conversation for the day.

"Oh, also did you make sure there is room in the parking lot for the buses? We don't have a designated area so I want to make sure they can park somewhere."

"Yes."

"You're the best."

"I know." Daisy smiled as we walked to the front gate.

The school buses arrived, and children rushed into the zoo giving the teachers barely enough time to do a head count. I was filled with excitement as I welcomed them to the zoo. Greeting the teacher, we shared enthusiasm for the day ahead, eager to showcase our diverse array of animals and their habitats.

As we discussed the itinerary, the teacher emphasized the importance of incorporating discussions about conservation efforts into the tour. I assured them that conservation was a priority for us, and I was eager to share our commitment to protecting endangered species with the students. With a shared passion for education and environmental stewardship, we set out to make the day a memorable and enlightening experience for all.

Daisy came to take over and guided all of the groups to the stations she had set up at the picnic area.

"Hi, my name is Daisy, I am the events coordinator." she confidently shook the teachers' hands.

The teacher smiled as Daisy went over all of the information she had laid out. She seemed very impressed with all that Daisy did being so young.

"I have groups set out based on the information you sent me. I made goody bags for students that included the itinerary, a map, as well as homemade animal trading cards. We have lunch at 12:30 as well."

Watching Daisy guide these students around and seeing their eyes wide open at the amazing animals was so heartwarming. It reminded me of when I was a child, and my dad would take me to the zoo. It's where I found my love for animals. I sat in the main circle watching students find their love for animals just like I did. I didn't think about my cancer, I thought about youth and the innocence of all of these children. Soon enough it was lunch.

Daisy and I met up and walked over to lunch. As we were walking over Daisy discussed the rest of the day. I was watching the children running around, innocently stirring their imaginations as they explored all of the animal exhibitions.

"Okay, so they have lunch until 1:15 and then there's a group presentation in the-" Daisy paused as she saw I wasn't paying attention at all. "Are you listening to anything I say?"

"I want children." I interjected.

Daisy hesitated not knowing what to say. I assumed it wasn't her problem, but she wanted to listen, so I decided to dump my traumas onto her.

"Really, it's not your problem, I don't want to burden you." I assured her.

"You can have children eventually; you just might be a little older." she innocently said to me.

"No… even if I do survive, I still will never be able to have children of my own. I have a tumor baby invading my uterus, I would never be able to breastfeed, and my ovaries are shot. I don't even get a period anymore." I explained to her.

"I'm sorry… there's always adoption." she offered.

"There is, isn't there?" I said as I pondered that possibility.

"Yeah, I was adopted," she said.

"Really? I didn't know that." I said.

"Yeah, my biological parents were drug addicts, and I was born going through withdrawal from heroin. I was adopted right out of the hospital because the cops wouldn't let me go home with them. It's honestly the best thing that's happened to me." she explained to me.

"Wow... Good to know. I'm glad everything worked out for you." I said to her.

She didn't seem too affected by it. I knew her adoptive parents and they were incredible, so it was understandable that she was more than satisfied. Despite not being biologically related, her adoptive parents have created an unbreakable bond with her, providing unwavering support, guidance, and affection. Their selflessness and devotion have shaped Daisy into the confident, resilient individual she is today, proving family is defined not by blood, but by the love and care shared between them.

Wanting to have a biological child was a deeply personal desire, rooted in the desire for a genetic connection and the experience of pregnancy and childbirth. However, grappling with the possibility of passing down genetic cancer always haunted me. It's a delicate balance between the desire for biological connection and the responsibility of ensuring a healthy start for future generations. Adoption remained a beautiful alternative; it gave me Daisy.

"As dark as it sounds, it will work out. If you live, you can adopt a child and raise them here to love animals. If you die. Your legacy will always be here, and you won't be in pain. You can look down from heaven and watch over all of these animals. Plus, you can haunt all the people who threw trash and human food in the enclosures." she said to me.

"I love you, Daisy." I said, smiling through tears.

"Love you too..." she said.

"Okay, let's go see this presentation you have set up."

"Oh, you'll love it, I found someone to let the kids pet the alligators!"

"What a great idea!"

"Don't worry, they're nice alligators."

"Oh great, nice alligators, I'll let Florida know to train their gators better."

"Please do, one ate a grandma just last week!"

"Oh dear!"

The zookeeper, clad in khaki, strolled confidently into the classroom, an old projector humming at his side. He captured the imaginations of the fourth graders with tales of alligator antics. With each fact shared, his passion for these prehistoric predators ignited the room, turning curious minds into budding reptile enthusiasts. Through vivid imagery and captivating stories, he unveiled the mysteries of the alligator kingdom, leaving the students wide-eyed and eager for more. Amidst his presentation, he brought out a surprise—a pet alligator named Snappy—for the kids to see up close. With jaws dropped, the students marveled at the sight, their fascination with the little guy growing with each passing moment. Daisy and I watched as each student went to pet Snappy, all of them infatuated with their encounter.

The alligator presentation quickly wrapped up and the students began to group together on the bus. I watched Daisy help the teachers make sure nothing was left behind or nothing was missing on our end. She amazed me, between preparing the say and executing it beautifully.

Daisy wasn't just my assistant or events coordinator as she terms it. She was like the little sister I never had. Growing up an only child, I didn't have someone to confide in or a young nag to bother me all the time. Although she was five years younger than me. I still related to her and told her everything.

~

Henry walked in as we were cleaning up. Children's maps and drops of ice cream were scattered throughout the park. He seemed exhausted from work but was entertained by how much we had to do. He noticed how our mess was so similar to a middle school.

"It looks like a tornado came through here."

Henry laughed, surveying the papers and scraps of food scattered about.

"Kind of, a bunch of fourth graders were here on a field trip." Daisy replied.

"How did that go?" he asked her.

"Great, can't you tell?" I smiled.

"I guess so, they clearly had fun!" he replied.

As we strolled to the salad place for dinner, I couldn't shake the pressing thought on my mind. With each step, my heart pounded louder, until finally, I mustered the courage to broach the subject. Amidst the bustling street, I gently turned to Henry, my words tentative yet determined. I spoke of dreams and uncertainties, of hopes for a future that seemed elusive.

With salads in hand, we walked together, discussing the possibility of children, our voices intermingling with the city's rhythm. In that fleeting moment, amidst the mundane task of figuring our what to add to our salads, we delved into the depths of our shared aspirations, navigating the delicate balance between longing and acceptance of the cloudiness of my possibility to have children. Yet, an unspoken truth lingered between us, the cruel reality of cancer casting a shadow over our dreams of parenthood.

Despite our shared desire for children, Henry hesitated at the mention of adoption. He expressed concerns about the complexities and uncertainties that came with it, revealing a reluctance to embrace an alternative path to parenthood. His reservations stemmed not from a lack of love or desire, but from a deeply ingrained hope for a biological connection seemed unattainable.

As we continued our conversation his apprehension became palpable, casting a sobering light on our shared dreams. While we were sitting and dining on the corner, we continued to ponder on our options to have a family. Amidst the uncertainties, our bond remained steadfast, a beacon of support and understanding in the face of adversity.

My husband meant well amidst all of his prickly demeanor. I understood his desire for children, a tangible legacy to cherish in my abs. However, I was unable to fulfill this wish, cancer took our desire for children away. Thus, I was compelled to exert every effort to prolong my life, to remain a steadfast presence for him to cling to in times of need.

~

Before I left for the day, I noticed Daisy struggling with a visitor. It didn't seem to be a bad struggle, more so a confusing struggle. I walked over to them and asked what was going on. Daisy explained that this family only spoke Spanish, but we were not prepared for that. Daisy also only knows Italian and classical Latin because of her musical background. She tried her hardest to help by speaking Italian, but it wasn't the best.

"Hola, coma esta? Estoy aquí para ayudar!" I replied

"Muchas gracias!"

"A mis hijos les encantan los anómalos, pero es difícil que todos sean ingleses."

"Entiendo. ¡sígueme!"

I guided this family through the zoo and translated all of the exhibits to the best of my ability. Daisy called Henry to tell him I would be late so that he didn't worry my health wasn't tanking. It only took me an hour to bring them all through the zoo. I also gave the children a little behind-the-scenes so they could meet some animals up close. The little girls were so fascinated with the baby cubs while the young boy's day was made when I let him hold an alligator.

"Since when do you know Spanish?!" Daisy asked me, surprised

"I did a study abroad in Spain in college and I guess I just picked it up quickly from Latin." I explained to her.

"Huh that's cool, never knew that about you!" She replied

"I'm full of surprises!" I smiled "But seriously though, because you have Italian and Latin under your belt, you'll be able to speak any language"

"I think I'll stick to my classical languages for piano"

I left for home after my little tour of the zoo and was met with Henry cooking dinner. As soon as I walked into the door, I could smell the spiciness of the tacos he was crafting together. His school had a half day, so he had the privilege of going to the store to pick up different ingredients. Of course, he decided to choose a spicy meal that I knew my stomach couldn't handle so he cooked me my own tacos that consisted of plain meat and lettuce.

Chapter 14

Henry and I sat on the couch, having our nightly date of Law and Order and popcorn. He was working on the computer while I was deeply invested in the dark plot of the episode.

"Hey, I have a huge favor to ask of you and you can absolutely say no" Henry said to me

"What is it?" I asked concerningly

"Would you be able to substitute teach for me tomorrow?" he asked

"I mean I don't know what to do?" I said

"It's okay, you're just going to basically babysit and keep everyone in line." he assured me

"I guess I can" I hesitantly accepted

"Great thank you!" he smiled and kissed my forehead

"Wait, where do I go, what do I do with them? You've told me nothing" I said to him as he rushed to try and get to his meeting on time. I had no information on what to do and he didn't have time to explain.

"Don't worry, just talk to the front desk, they'll direct you and show you where to go. The teacher left sub notes and an assignment, it's senior biology so you'll be fine." he said walking out the door

"Oh okay, that'll work" I said

"Exactly! See you at school!" he smiled

"See you there" I said

I was excited to go teach biology. Well not teach but kind of teaching. I could share all that I learned in college as I literally graduated with a degree in biology.

I walked to the front desk. Noticing Vera was not on that day. A woman sat at Vera's desk, I had never seen her before, but she was very kind. Very different from Vera's cold attitude towards life.

"Hi, I'm here to substitute teach" I said

"Oh, we don't have you in the roster" the woman said looking very confused.

"My husband is Mr. Williams. He asked me to come in this morning" I said, handing over my ID.

"Oh, ok then…I'll show you the way" she smiled "So, there are 5 classes she has, all biology except for one anatomy class. Mrs. Burns left out some assignments for them to do. If they get finished just let them talk quietly." she explained to me

"Sounds easy enough" I replied

"Here you are… good luck" she said as she quickly walked away.

My nerves heightened considering she wished me luck to just watch a class. I honestly had no clue what to expect. The assignments seemed easy enough and I could definitely help with them.

"So, you're the Mrs. Williams, Mr. Williams always talks about" I heard from the doorframe.

I turned to see another teacher standing in the doorway, he came from the classroom across the hall.

"He talks about me?" I laughed

"Yea its annoying" he joked

"Oh ok... I'll let him know" I replied

"I'm just kidding…let me know if you need any help! Mr. Jones, by the way." he said to me before walking back to his classroom.

"Do you guys have sex or is Mr. Williams as boring in bed as he is in school" a student yelled as they all began to fill the seats from the hallway.

"Inappropriate Miss Miller!" Mr. Jones yelled from across the hall after hearing.

I knew it was going to be a long day after dealing with teenage hormones, bullies, and making sure the quiet kids don't get swallowed alive.

The bell rang and most students were in, except for a couple of stragglers who had no care they were late for class. I ignored the late students as I didn't want to press any more buttons.

"So, guys I can help you with anything on these assignments. I have my degree in biology, so I've been through all of this" I smiled

I continued to hand everything out and noticed students were less than enthusiastic to do the simple worksheet that was assigned.

"I'm not doing this" one student argued

"Well, I'm pretty sure it's a grade" I replied

"Don't care, I'm not going it" she repeated in a more agitated tone

"Okay I'll let Mrs. Burns know" I said trying to diminish the situation

"No, you won't. You'll do it for me" she said

"I'm sorry I can't do that" I replied

"Yes, you can, or I'll rip those tumors out myself" she yelled angrily

I didn't want to anger her anymore, so I grabbed a seasoned teacher to help me. "Mr. Jones!"

"Grace! Office now!" he yelled storming into the classroom

"Screw you… go to hell" she said as she ran to the office

"I'm so sorry about that!" He said

He assured me it wouldn't happen again. He claimed that was the only student who would cause problems.

"No, it's okay, I don't know how you guys do this" I said "If I was talking like that at 13 years old my mom would have kicked me out of the house before I even finished the sentence"

"You get used to it I guess," he said, "it definitely helps you grow a pair!"

"Oh, I can see why!" I laughed "Please tell me Mrs. Burns will be back tomorrow"

"Oh, yea she will, she just had some appointment with her kid she forgot about." he assured me

"Okay good because I think this will be a one-and-done situation" I said confidently

"Trust me, I get it!" he said as he walked back to his classroom.

I went through the day with constant bullying for being married to a teacher. It didn't hurt, it honestly was kind of funny hearing how creative kids can get with insults but can't even sit down to write a paper in one sitting.

"Hey, how's it going?" Henry asked as he casually walked into the classroom.

"They hate you!" I said to him

He was the one who disciplined the student who yelled at me but didn't tell me anything about what happened to her.

"Oh, I know, I'm surprised I haven't gotten shanked yet!" he said ever so casually

"Why are they like this?" I asked

"When I came in this school was a mess, disciplinary wise, so I came and changed everything around. They were so used to the old disciplinarian letting them do anything they want and that just doesn't fly with me" he explained

"That makes sense." I said

I began to pack up my things and I asked him to help me organize the paperwork for Mrs. burns.

"You know me, you can't get anything past me!" he said, smiling and grouping all of the assignments based on periods.

He asked who was in charge of the zoo that day since I was away helping him. I told him Daisy was in charge for the day. He thought I was crazy for letting a 19-year-old in charge, but I think I made the right choice. She was very mature and had an entrepreneur's mindset.

"Will we see a lion crossing the street on our way home?" he joked as we headed to the subway to ride home.

"A lion strolling the avenue of the Americas? That would be something!" I laughed

Daisy somehow managed to keep all animals alive and enclosed which both Henry and I were very surprised about. I knew I now had someone who could manage when I was in chemo or just too sick to go in. It was relieving to know I could trust her.

~

We were walking home, navigating the bustling world of Manhattan. We headed to the subway and took the six train up to Harlem and then took the five home to The Bronx. It wasn't an easy trip, but it was what we did to afford living.

The subway held a diverse tapestry of human differences and indifferences with each passing stop. Amidst the rhythmic hum of the train and the flickering lights, I find myself immersed in a silent symphony of stories. Faces, each one a chapter waiting to be explored, paint the canvas of the subway car.

From the weary commuter lost in thought to the animated conversations of friends, each moment offers a glimpse into the intricate web of human existence. As the train hurtles through tunnels, I watch as passengers board and deboard. They all have different stops, different lives, different stories in the grand narrative of urban life.

"So, I was wondering what your plan was for when I'm gone" I asked him as we got off the train and began our walk home.

"If" he stopped me before I could start another sentence.

"Oh, stop with the if and when, I'm dying and I'm not getting out of this." I argued

"So, what do you mean by my plan" he asked

We pushed our way through the bustling streets. It was hard to get such a serious conversation in, but we managed.

"What's your plan for your future without me?" I asked.

We continued to walk home at rush hour. Everyone had the same plan which made it difficult to hold a conversation let alone keep up with Henry rushing home.

"Well, if you must ask, I don't know if I'll remarry or anything. Not sure what I'll do with your zoo." he said

He fumbled with his keys. Shuffling through his school keys to find our house key.

"I want you to remarry though" I said as I watched him. "Maybe you should separate personal and school keys?"

"I've got it" he said "I don't think I can remarry"

I said to him. "Hen, you are 25 years old. You have a whole life ahead of you, you can't just stop for me."

I stopped him from unpacking his bags and decompressing from work to continue our conversation. I was so tired of him always avoiding deep conversations, especially about me. I never liked having those conversations, but I knew I needed to because I had to get my affairs in order. My time was limited, not his.

"We've been together for years, that's a long time, all of my teenage life, your teen life and childhood. You were my first love and I believe you are my last" he replied

Tears pooled in my eyes, "I love you and I love you to death but to my death, not yours. You can't stop your life at 26 years old. You have to move on but without forgetting me." I said

I pulled my ring off my hand for once and showed it to him, having it be put on a chain. I didn't want him to bury my wedding ring in the ground for it to just rot away with me. I wanted him to keep pour physical bond as strong as our emotional bond.

"My wedding ring… when I die, I want you to take it and wear it as a necklace, I know that is a little girly, but It'll keep me close to your heart."

He quickly put it back on my hand and held back tears. Henry was not the kind of man to cry a lot, so this was a rare moment we had.

"I really can't do this" he said

"How do you think I feel" I laughed trying to make a lighter view of the situation

"You have the easy part; I have to go on and live without you" he said

"I guess dying is the easy part, isn't it" I said as I walked over to the window.

Watching the birds nibbling at the bird feeder. The First thing I bought when we moved to New York.

"Well, I just have to go to sleep, and I get to watch over you. I'm not going anywhere"

The bird reminded me of the zoo and how I can't let it be given up on again and I needed to be assured He wouldn't just let it go to shambles. I knew he wasn't a fan of the whole situation.

"What's your plan for the zoo, it's been abandoned once, I can't see it being abandoned again." I asked him

"I promise you; I will keep it going, it will continue to thrive, and you will see it be as amazing as you left it. Maybe even better" he said as he joined me at the window

"I need a will" I said to him

"I guess you do…" he said solemnly

"Yeah, I will leave the zoo to your name, but I don't want you to give up your life for it. I think Daisy will be fine to follow my lead." I said

"Well, I can still help out and everything" he said to me

"Absolutely but I don't want you to quit your job and everything so having Daisy will help" I said confidently

"Okay, I mean I wasn't planning on doing that, but I will make sure it is well staffed, and Daisy is never leaving."

"Are we kidnapping Daisy?" He asked with a smile on his face

"We are kidnapping Daisy" I laughed

"We discussed this with no one!" We laughed as we watched the birds together.

I wrote up an informal will so that if I were to get hit by a bus or something, it was there. I knew I had to eventually go to an attorney, but I just was not emotionally ready for it.

Chapter 15

Everyone loves birthdays, my birthday happened to be a somber time for me. 24 years old, I would probably be celebrating my last birthday to celebrate. What a great thing to say!

It's weird to think next year I could not exist. Well obviously, I exist but not in physical form. I was so worked up and distracted by my cancer that I honestly forgot about my birthday was quickly approaching. Henry was excited, he loved celebrating birthdays and making them a huge deal, but I didn't want to anything. I wanted to just skip that day without anyone mentioning it.

After awhile, people would see my birthday and think about how I was dying, and no one cared about the fact I celebrate my birthday every year. My birthday slowly became synonymous with my impending death. Everyone was so kind and bent over backwards for me, not to celebrate my life, but to aid me and my family when I'm sick…which is always.

Henry kissed me as I slowly woke up, "Good morning, happy birthday sweetheart!"

"Morning…" I replied quietly. I still wasn't fully awake and was not in the mood to go celebrate.

"What's wrong, it's a great day!" He said

Knowing he wasn't going to stop the conversation, I decided to get up. "No, its not, its just any other day because we are not doing anything" I said

"Of course we are silly. It's your birthday!" He said kissing me on the forehead.

"I really don't need to do anything" I assured him

"Why not?" He asked

"Because its my last birthday and I don't want this to be a celebration of my death and that's what its going to turn into" I explained to him.

"Okay well, let's not think that its your least because it may not be!" He said, sitting on the bed with me. "What if we go out, just the two of us and there is one rule!"

"And what is that?" I asked

"We are not allowed to say the c-word" he replied

I watched as he got dressed for work and I grabbed my bathrobe and glasses. We headed downstairs and Henry brewed coffee in his travel mug and poured me some in my mug from the hospital gift shop.

"Ok but what if I get sick or need help up the stairs" I asked

"You mean what if you get carsick or have troubles rom recovering from knee surgery?" He said

"Great...now I'm lying so I'll get a nice fast pass to hell" I laughed

"I think God can forgive you for this one instance. Besides I'll take the blame" he smiled as he got ready for work.

"Fine..." I said, reluctantly, "when will you be home and where are we going?"

"Don't sound so excited!" he laughed "I'll be home by 4 and it'll be a surprise, I'll help you get ready!"

"Wait…what do you mean help me?" I asked him before he left

"Relax… I mean I'll help you find something to wear!" He laughed

"Ok… deal…nothing to fancy please, I can't do heels anymore!" I added

"Flats can be sexy too!" He said, walking out the door.

"Yea yea yea!" I said as he left for work.

I wasn't planning on doing anything for my birthday, but Henry had plans to make it a whole big day. While I didn't plan anything, I didn't want to stay home and sulk in my own bed. I left to go got the zoo, I didn't want to work but I wanted to hang out with the animals. I knew they wouldn't treat me any differently because I was ill, and they wouldn't bother me with different crap that I didn't care about. All anyone wanted to do was mentioned how sickly I was and how if I needed anything, don't hesitate to ask. The great thing about animals is they can't talk!

As I walked into the zoo, I saw daisy holding a bottle of champagne, two glasses, and a bundle of 'happy Birthday' balloons. I walked over to her, and she opened wide for a big hug. She wished me best wishes and we sat at the table next to the elephants.

"Thanks for this" I smiled

"I thought you could use a nice day out" she replied.

I sipped my champagne, "You have no idea"

"Well, the zoo has been doing well and everything is running beautifully" she said

"Awesome! Thank you so much for your help, I know I've thrown a lot of you and quite frankly, I really wasn't expecting to do that" I said sincerely

"Oh no you're fine! Ive been having so much fun and it's honestly been a nice break from all the strictness of school. You have no idea how boring it can be to sit through a three-hour class listening to different 100-year-old pieces to "tune" your ears"

"That's crazy! What other classes do you have to take? Is it all music or any liberal arts classes?"

"They're all piano, music, or music history classes but I am taking one Political science class"

"Oh, that's good! I like that, then you're not wasting your money on useless classes like astronomy or something"

"Yea its nice, but it could be nice to have change of pace though"

"That's true but your spending money on something that's meaningful, imagine spending $60,000 to take a class on British literature when you're getting a degree in biology!"

"Yea I get that! But on the other hand, it's tiring to only be taking the same classes, so I feel like college is a lose lose."

"A college degree is far from a lose lose, and Juilliard?! You have a ticket to New York!"

"Your right but I don't know, Im not sure what I want to do at this point"

"Listen... a year ago I was supposed to be here in vet school, but here I am, a zoo owner, a cancer patient, and a best friend to my estranged niece"

"Cheers to change!"

"Amen!"

We clinked champagne glasses and continued to talk about life. I loved having someone ignore my cancer and just talk to me like a normal person. Daisy managed that beautifully. I was so grateful to her for holding herself so well while dealing with everything I've thrown at her. The last thing I expected was for a nineteen-year-old to be the most understanding of my situation. My whole life was thrown upside down and leave it to my tiny niece to help me pick up the pieces in the most normal fashion.

~

While this was my most abnormal birthday, I wanted something that felt as normal as possible. Henry had planned a small dinner at a big restaurant where we would blend in and no one would notice us, which was exactly what I wanted. Surrounded by the hum of conversations and clinking of silverware to the plates, we were just another table celebrating an ordinary evening. The dim lighting and cozy ambiance provided a comforting anonymity, allowing us to share laughter and stories without a single mention of my diagnosis overshadowing the moment. Even when I had to excuse myself to quietly throw up in the restroom, no one in the restaurant seemed to care or notice. For a few precious hours, amidst the bustling crowd, we reclaimed a sense of normalcy, savoring the simple joy of being together.

Living in New York City offered a unique and liberating anonymity that was invaluable during my battle with cancer. In the vast, bustling metropolis, I was just another person navigating the vibrant streets, blending into the sea of people all living completely different lives. The city's inherent diversity and constant motion let me to live my life without the constant reminders of my illness. Strangers on the subway, baristas at the corner café, and fellow pedestrians treated me like anyone else, free from the weight of pity or special treatment. This sense of normalcy provided a comforting escape, enabling me to focus on the moments of joy and connection the city had to offer. In NYC, I found the freedom to be myself, to live each day without being defined by my diagnosis.

While Henry had it an incredibly normal night, I couldn't help but feel discouraged by all of the simple things I took advantage of prior to being sick. I wanted to drink so much I could forget all of my problems. I wanted to go home and have the best birthday sex with my husband. Instead, I got to be hungover without a single drop of alcohol. We tried to be intimate, but I quickly realized pain and embarrassment would end that. Henry tried but nothing he could say or cover, wouldn't stop my dark feelings from overcoming our entire relationship.

I stopped him out of frustration, feeling that I couldn't feel myself getting in the mood to have sex. "Im sorry"

"Why are you sorry? Its not your fault" he replied

"No but it is, I know I can't help it, but I feel bad" I said, pulling away and grabbing the covers.

"Don't, we don't need to have sex to have a great night. We can watch some TV" he said

"Were both naked right now and I know that you are currently excited" I lightly laughed

"So? I can get it down and we can just watch TV and have a nice evening of..." he turned the TV on to immediately see the discovery channel and two animals mating. "Ok we are not going to watch this…"

"See even the animals get sex and not me!"

"Stop… I don't want to laugh but you're making me laugh and I feel bad!" He said with a hidden smirk on his face.

"Henry we are sitting in bed, naked, your hard, and I'm dry because my body decided to reject my happiness. Its funny!" I bursted into laughter

"Your weird" he laughed "well, happy birthday!"

"Let's watch those animals" I joked

"Is that the type of porn you're into?" He laughed

I nudged him, grabbing the remote from his hand to change the channel, "Shut up! Your gross!"

"You're the one who's the animal enthusiast!"

We sat and talked more, it turned into a better night rather than if we did end up having sex or getting drunk. Also, as a plus, I didn't get sick at all. It was the most normal night I had in a long time.

~

It was a daunting task to work with daisy to keep the zoo alive but being with animals has been such a privilege. Reviving the failing zoo requires a concerted effort fueled by passion and innovation. With a vision for revitalization, dedicated caretakers and conservationists collaborate to breathe new life into the once-forgotten sanctuary.

Through strategic partnerships with local communities and businesses, the zoo's mission is redefined, emphasizing education, conservation, and immersive experiences. Dilapidated enclosures are transformed into vibrant habitats, carefully curated to mimic the natural environments of the animals they house. Innovative conservation programs engage visitors of all ages, fostering a deeper appreciation for wildlife and habitat preservation. As word spreads of the zoo's resurgence, crowds flock once more to its gates, eager to witness the transformation firsthand. With each step forward, the zoo emerges as a beacon of hope, demonstrating the power of collective action in safeguarding our planet's precious biodiversity.

"I have chemo at noon so you will be in charge after that" I said to Daisy as she prepared for the day ahead.

"Got it" she replied

"Thank you, I seriously appreciate all of your help!" I said sincerely to her.

"Of course!" She smiled

As we were beginning our day, I brought up the conversation of the zoo being run by her once I was gone. I didn't want to bring the mood down, but I needed to know she was able to take on such a daunting task. She hugged me intensely as tears welled in her eyes. Without using words, she overwhelmingly accepted.

"Don't cry, no need to cry." I said smiling

"But you're dying, and I don't know I just feel guilty I guess" she said

"No, absolutely do not feel guilty at all. This is my choice, and I can't change what's going on. I can only focus on keeping my affairs in order which includes this zoo." I explained "I am confident that you can handle this, and I will make sure you are completely prepared."

"Thank you…" she said

"You are welcome, thank you" I replied "I'm going to go feed the lions"

I walked to the lion enclosure and made sure to say hello to each animal as I passed. I remember reading somewhere that animals could sense cancer. I guess humans with cancer release a different smell only animals can smell. It was fascinating to think animals could know someone has cancer before anyone else does. If only they can show a clear-cut warning a sign.

"I'm going to miss you guys the most, don't tell the others though!" I said to them

I made sure to give them food and water and stayed to play a little. As I was throwing dead meat carcasses, I saw a young girl watching from a distance. She was watching me feed the lion cubs and I could tell she had a peeked interest.

"Hi, sweetie!" I yelled from the enclosure

"Hello" a quiet little voice said

"Would you like to feed a lion?" I asked as I pointed to the baby cub sitting in the small hut

Her face lit up as I brought a young cub over.

"This is Dana, she was born about a month ago. Her favorite food is berries, would you like to feed her?"

"Does she bite?" She asked, hesitant to pet her.

I assured her the cub was very sweet and offered her some berries to give to her. As we were feeding the baby, I heard an angry yell from afar.

"Samantha, you need to stop running off! We talked about this!" her mother said with a sigh of relief. "I'm so sorry, I will make sure she doesn't do this again"

"No, a problem, we were just saying hi to miss Dana" I assured the panicking mother

"Mommy, look I fed a lion" she smiled

"Ok sweetie, it's time to go, we need to go wash our hands"

The mother grabbed her daughter's hand and tried to coax her to continue on with their day.

"But I was playing!" The daughter protested

"Dana will be here, don't worry! Go ahead and grab lunch, I think Dana is ready for her nap" I said

I tried to help the mother with her reluctant daughter who wants to play with every animal there.

"Thank you!" The mother smiled as they headed to the cafeteria.

I put the cub back and ran to Daisy to talk to her about a plan. I was out of breath from not being able to rush anywhere. I tried to catch my breath as Daisy offered me a seat. I declined, not wanting to be a victim. I always tried to ignore symptoms, but these became so overwhelming I slowly came to realize that this was not like any other symptom I've had before.

"So, I think we should have a petting zoo section" I said to her, still unable to catch my breath fully.

"With which animals" she asked

"I mean obviously the nice ones, but I think giving kids the opportunity to pet a monkey or a llama would be so fun!" I said

"You're right! That would be fun" she said happily, while still worried about me. "You really don't sound good"

"No no I'm fine, I swear" I said, "I have to go because I have chemo in a half hour."

As I was sitting in my office, getting everything ready so I could leave. The room began to spin, it continued to speed up. I ignored it and tried to go on with my day, refusing to tell Daisy. I knew something was up, but I didn't want to upset daisy. I'm genuinely thought I could get home without disturbing anyone, but I was clearly wrong...

Daisy sensed something was off as I wasn't my usual self. "Do you need a ride?" She asked me.

"Umm yea I think so" I said as I thought I couldn't make it on the subway.

"Okay, lets go" she said, she knew I was not okay, and I needed someone to help me.

We left for the hospital as I felt myself losing consciousness. I felt really weak and dizzy, and I just couldn't get myself to focus on string words.

The constant throbbing in my head felt like a relentless drumbeat echoing through my skull. My vision swamped, the world around me dancing in a blurry haze. Strange moments of uncontrollable jerking and twitching in my body left me terrified. My limbs were heavy as if dragging through molasses. It was a sensation I wouldn't wish on anyone—a constant reminder of the invisible battle raging inside me. A deep, throbbing pain that would not go away no matter what.

The pain consumed my entire body. I was gasping for breath as Daisy ran into the hospital for help.

I kept asking for Henry, but I couldn't form coherent sentences. I kept panicking as doctors swarmed around me, their faces a blur of concern and determination. They ordered a barrage of tests—MRI, CT scans, blood work—all in an urgent attempt to unravel the mystery within my brain. Needles pricked my skin, machines hummed and whirred, and I felt like a mere pawn in the intricate chess game of my health. Each test brought a glimmer of hope mixed with dread, the anticipation of answers mingling with the fear of what they might reveal. As the minutes stretched into hours, I clung to the belief that somewhere in the midst of all these tests there would be a light at the end of the tunnel.

"Henry? Hey, where are you?" Daisy called in a panic.

"I'm at work, what's going on?" Henry answered unsuspectingly.

"Philomena in the ER, I don't know what's going on. They won't tell me because I'm not family. I-" she replied, barely able to get her words out as she filled with anxiety.

"I'm on my way." he said.

He dropped his phone, leaving all of his belongings behind. Racing through Manhattan in the quickest possible ways. He maneuvered every car that sat on FDR drive. Beeping at all of the car distracted by their phones, acting like sheep who slowly wait for each car to take their time, as though they have never been to New York. Slowly, they all took in all of the views they can see from the main highway of the city. It seemed as through he was the only native on the road at the time, all the other cars were taking their time to take in what's around them.

After daisy arrived, it was all a blur for me. I don't remember anything except our arrival. I wasn't scared but I wasn't afraid. I didn't know how to feel. I just felt numb, nothing, I don't remember anything that happened from when I left the zoo to a few days after.

When Henry arrived, he frantically looked for answered from each front desk he went to. No nurses had definitive answers as I was still in surgery at the time. Finally, a neurosurgeon came out to speak with next of kin, which just consisted of Henry alone, plus Daisy. My dad was not aware of anything. Henry didn't want to worry him, thinking it wasn't a huge deal since Daisy didn't really explain the full story. She left out the seizure in the ER, the major emergency surgery, as well as other things, when talking over the phone.

The Doctors explained to him that the cancer had spread to my brain. I was rushed into surgery to try and remove the tumor, but the outcome did not look great. The cancer eventually invaded my entire body, I was owned by tumors. There was no turning back after this point.

"What happened?" He asked every nurse in an angry panic.

"I have no clue…we were at the zoo, and she just started gasping for breath, then she couldn't form full sentences and I just don't know what happened. Did I do something?" Daisy said

She was trying to assure him she would be ok while still feeling herself panic, anxiety eating her away with each passing minute I was in surgery.

In the waiting room, Henry's anxiety was palpable as he sat, his heart heavy with worry, waiting for news of my brain surgery. Time seemed to stretch endlessly, each passing minute feeling like an eternity.

The silence was oppressive, broken only by the rhythmic ticking of the clock on the wall. Every sound, every footstep echoing down the corridor, made him jump, his nerves frayed with anticipation. He prayed fervently for the skilled hands of the surgeons and the comforting embrace of good news to envelop them soon.

Beside him, Daisy sat, offering quiet support in the midst of the tense atmosphere. They exchanged worried glances and whispered words of encouragement, their bond strengthening in the face of adversity.

Together, they navigated the agonizing wait, finding solace in each other's presence amidst the uncertainty. As they waited for news, Henry found a sliver of comfort knowing he was not alone in his apprehension. In that shared moment of vulnerability, their unlikely friendship became an anchor, grounding them amidst the storm of emotions swirling around them.

As the doctor emerged from the operating room with a reassuring smile, announcing the success of the surgery, a sense of relief flooded the waiting room.

However, the doctor's next words tempered their elation—there was a long road ahead for the recovery from brain surgery. Despite the success of the procedure, the journey to full recovery would be challenging and require patience and resilience. Henry and Daisy exchanged a glance, their expressions reflecting a mixture of gratitude for the positive outcome and determination to support me through the difficult days ahead. They knew while the surgery marked a significant milestone, it was just the beginning of a journey fraught with uncertainty and obstacles. Together, they resolved to stand by my side, offering unwavering support and encouragement as I embarked on the arduous road to recovery.

Chapter 16

I remember waking up with a throbbing headache, my husband by my side, and my dad there. I couldn't speak. All I could do was watch and figure out how to communicate with my eyes. I kept panicking thinking I'd never be able to talk or walk or live again. I felt I was going to be confined to a bed for the rest of my short life, the sensation of a tube down my throat and the rhythmic hum of the ventilator adding to my discomfort.

Both Henry and my dad were by my side, they continuously comforted me, assuring me everything would be okay. Henry held my hand as my dad stroked the side of my face.

I found myself locked in a relentless debate, questioning whether the struggle of being alive was worth enduring. All I craved was relief from the ceaseless pain, the relentless suffering, and the suffocating blanket of sadness that enveloped me. The stabbing sensation in my throat and the pounding hammer in my brain tortured me relentlessly, pushing me to the brink of despair. Each moment felt like an eternity of agony, and the overwhelming desire to escape it all consumed me. I wanted the torment to cease, yearning for peace to finally embrace me, even if it meant embracing death.

I thought I had a whole life ahead of me. I wanted to become a veterinarian, start a family with my husband, I wanted to grow old and retire at the beach. I knew this would never happen as my life was stripped from me so quickly, I couldn't even imagine my future anymore. It all became a distant memory will never become true. Like a dream, a little girl wants to become a pop star or a little boy who wants to play pro-football. It's possible but the reality of it actually happening slowly diminishes as life goes on. Everyone tries to tell you it's possible and that you just need to fight for your dreams but in reality, it won't ever happen, and parents know that. Only 1.6 percent of college football players make it pro but almost every child dreams of it.

Three months ago, my odds of beating this cancer were 80%, I am now at a 10% survival rate. I always wondered what happened. Was I too slow? Did I do something wrong? Did I wrong God? How did I go from 80 to 10 in only a few months… my health jumped off a cliff, along with my life and my plans for my future. It is the worst feeling in the world.

I watched as Henry paced the room and my dad just kept staring at me, waiting for me to bounce back and go back to normal. Henry continued to ask the doctors how long it would take for me to wake up but all that was said was time will tell. He didn't understand why this was all happening, I remember him telling my dad it was a curse. It was funny because I thought how this could be a curse. What curse? What did we do? I couldn't imagine what horrible thing I did to deserve this. It was unfathomable to think that God could do this to someone as revenge.

As I laid on the ventilator, Henry remained steadfast at my side, offering comfort in every way could. He gently adjusted the tubes and wires, ensuring my comfort despite the insurmountable pain I was plagued with. With soft words and tender gestures, he conveyed his love and unwavering support, his touch a source of familiar comfort amidst the clinical surroundings.

Though I couldn't respond, Henry stayed close, his presence a silent promise of enduring devotion and care to the end of my days. Through the steady rhythm of the ventilator, he whispered words of hope and encouragement, reminding me I was not alone in my struggle.

"Hey sweetie, I brought you a blanket from home, I'm not sure if you were cold but I thought maybe you could have a piece of home" he said

"Do you think she can hear us?" He asked my dad

"I'm sure she can, I've read that people in a coma can- "he replied, quickly being cut off by my dad.

Without finishing his sentence, Henry immediately corrected him. "She's not in a coma"

"I know but if a coma patient can hear, I'm sure she can" he replied, trying not to anger him.

"What if she doesn't wake up?"

"She will… she will…"

"She's always been strong, and this is no exception. Her body just needs to rest."

The weight of the diagnosis crushed me as I realized cancer had invaded not just one, but multiple parts of my body. It started in my breast, spreading its tendrils to my lungs, ovaries, and bloodstream, and now it has reached my brain. Each new revelation felt like another blow, shattering the fragile hope I held onto with each treatment and prognosis. Yet, amidst the overwhelming despair, I found a flicker of resilience, a determination to fight with every ounce of strength I possessed.

"I hate this…" Henry said

"Me too" my dad replied

"Why does this need to happen to her? She won't even kill a cockroach in our apartment. Last week there was a spider in our bathroom, and she cried when I killed it. All she wants to do is take care of others and now I can barely hold it together to take care of her." Henry said

He paced the room watching as my lungs filled and rested, all controlled by a machine.

"You're doing great, do not pin this on yourself" my father said as he comforted him, trying to get him to relax.

"Have you thought about staying home with her?" He asked

"I have but she won't let me quit" Henry replied

"She needs you home" he said

"Don't you think I know that?!" Henry yelled

"No need to yell" he tried to calm him.

"Who's going to pay the bills? Who's going to pay the rent? She can't work!" He continued to rant in anger

"No, I know but you can file for unemployment, you can find help. I will help you" my dad suggested

"No, I'm not accepting handouts, Philomena would be so upset if we started taking handouts" he said

"Look she may not even make it out of this, if that's the case then we don't even need to worry about it!"

"She's going to make it, don't even think about that!" My dad said confidently as he guided Henry to a chair, trying to calm him down.

"I don't know…if not this time, it's going to come" he said teary eyed "you know she's asked about planning her funeral and will? How do I help her with that"

"She's got the easy part, dying is easy, it's what's left for us that's the difficult part." Henry added

"She's 23 years old… what 23-year-old has to plan their funeral"

"A lot unfortunately, she's joining the gruesome club of cancer"

"Just so fucking stupid" Henry said

He threw an empty water cup across the room in rage. The entire time he thought about all of the worse case scenarios.

The next day I woke up but still couldn't fully grasp what had happened. I was just laying in a daze as I watched everyone rushing around.

"Henry, why are you crying?" I asked in a dazed confusion. My voice raw and raspy from a tube's violent presence and exit.

Henry rushed to my side, a sigh of relief was let out when he saw I was awake and talking. "Hi Philomena, how are you feeling?" He asked.

"Hungry and tired and dizzy" I responded.

"Okay well you have a feeding tube in so you can't eat just yet, do you know where you are?" he replied

"Yes, I'm in the hospital" I said as a doctor came in to do routine vitals and bloodwork.

"Do you know how you got here" the doctor asked

"I remember Daisy taking me and then I just blacked out" I said

"Okay good, you had a craniotomy to remove a tumor in your parietal lobe. We got the entire thing, and you shouldn't need to worry too much about any side effects. Thankfully it was a very black and white surgery, and you should be able to go home and start physical therapy in a week or so." The doctor explained

I tried to get out of bed in a dazed state. I pulled all of the wires off and tried to pull the feeding tube out of my nose. "No no, I need to go home now" I said "Henry, you need to go to work, how's the animals? Is Daisy, okay?"

"See, I told you she'd be fine" my dad smiled

~

After another four days in the hospital, I was discharged, but the journey to recovery was far from over. It took several months of intensive therapy and rehabilitation to even begin to feel like myself again.

Yet, despite my progress, the memory of that life-altering brain surgery loomed large, casting a shadow over my once vibrant existence. I grappled with the realization I was now officially classified as handicapped, a label which weighed heavily on my spirit. The simplest tasks became monumental challenges, and the road ahead seemed hauntingly uncertain.

Navigating through physical therapy after brain surgery, I found comfort in the unwavering presence of Henry by my side. His steady support was a constant source of strength as I grappled with the challenges of rehabilitation. With each grueling session, he offered encouragement and reassurance, his belief in my ability to heal. Together, we faced the hurdles of recovery, his hand a reassuring anchor as I pushed through moments of doubt and exhaustion.

As we journeyed through the highs and lows of rehabilitation, his steadfast presence was a beacon of hope, guiding me towards a future filled with promise and possibility. From balance exercises to fine motor skill drills, Henry stood beside me, offering support through all of this, his presence infusing each session with an extra dose of determination and resilience.

The toll of chemotherapy was compounded by the lingering effects of my recent brain surgery. The treatments exacerbated the physical and emotional strain already present from the surgical intervention. The combination of chemotherapy's side effects and the delicate state of my recovering brain left me feeling drained and vulnerable. Navigating through the waves of nausea, fatigue, and cognitive fog was a daunting task, made all the more challenging by the ongoing recovery process. Despite the uphill battle, I drew strength from the support of my loved ones.

~

Every day was a new day when it came to dealing with Vera. She was like a sister I never had, but not in the way you would think. Every time she would come to talk to me it was a new dagger to my emotions and confidence. I built a wall between us so her constant insults and rudeness wouldn't bother me eventually.

This particular day, I heard a knock on the door and was surprised to see Vera at the door with a tray of baked lasagna. I was completely shocked by the act of kindness but extremely grateful, nonetheless.

"Vera? What brings you to this side of the wall?" I asked, standing at the door.

"I was just bringing this" she replied, holding a deliciously smelling tray of lasagna.

"No Berlin joke?" I laughed

"Nope, just lasagna!" she said

"Did my vera get kidnapped, where's mean vera?" I asked, being very hesitant. I was so confused as to why she was being so nice to me.

"Mean Vera retired… I have realized that you have a lot going on and maybe having some help would be nice. Plus, your husband always raves about my lasagna at work so it's a win win." She replied

"Well… thank you… would you like to come in?" I said, still confused.

"If you would like?" she replied

"Seriously, what happened to Vera" I said, welcoming her into my living room.

Vera came inside and we began to talk about life, her past, and everything in between. We began to discuss her ex-husband and my mother.

"Not to be that person, but may I ask what happened? Between you and your ex-husband?" I asked, hesitantly

"How'd, you know about that?" she asked, seeming surprised I knew anything about it.

"Oh, I just heard it from somewhere, don't really remember when or who?" I replied. I didn't want to rat out the bartender who told me because he really didn't go into detail.

"Well, my ex found a woman at his job, and they began a 3-year relationship behind my back. Little did I know, they had a child together, got engaged, and then planned to move across the country. All without telling me until the day before he left." She explained

"Jeez, I'm so sorry…" I said as I poured her another glass of wine

"It's okay, I guess it's good he's happy or whatever" she laughed

"But that's still so horrible!" I added

"Oh definitely, you can just never truly trust anyone." She said as she hinted at my wedding picture on the wall.

"I will say though, he was rich, so I got a decent alimony from the divorce."

"What did he do for a. Living?" I asked.

"He was a cardiologist, yet he still destroyed my heart. His way of saying sorry was to write a check." She added.

We continued to talk about life, and this was the one time we actually bonded, and it was truly a nice time. I wasn't expecting such a soft side to Vera, so I was delighting to have a small invite to her vulnerability.

"Well, if were going into our deep sides here, what happened between you and your mom?"

"What do you mean? She passed when I was 12 from lung disease"

"Yea but I just sense there's something there"

"I mean we didn't have a great relationship, but it was what it was."

"See, that's why. I never wanted kids. I never wanted to neglect or anything. Also, my ex left me for a kid, so I don't need to worry about anyone leaving me"

"Don't say that! I'm sure you'll find someone new eventually"

"Nah, I like the single life, I don't have to answer to anyone, or argue or anyone at home, its nice to be alone"

"Yea I guess but don't you get lonely?"

"Not at home, I have work to socialize, and home is my sanctuary"

"That makes sense, as long as your happy I guess" I replied, "It is nice when Henry's at work and I'm able to just lay in bed alone."

"See exactly, its great when your able to relax on your own and get the bed to yourself"

We ended our conversation with talking about the zoo. She talked to Henry about it at work and was still shocked by all of my hard work and dedication. It was exhausting but I told her it was all worth it.

"Before you go, can I ask you something?" I said before she let herself out.

"What's up?" She asked me

"Why did you come over?" I asked, "I know you wanted to bring me dinner and stuff but why did you really come over?" I replied

"I guess I just wanted to make peace. Your sick and I like your husband. I don't want to have you possibly die and live knowing I was nothing but an asshole to you" she explained

"So, you wanted to make amends before I die?" I said in a laughing, light tone.

"I wouldn't word it like that…" she smiled

"No, thank you, no one has accepted my reality so, to know that someone in my life has its comforting?" I explained

"Was that an insult?" She replied

"No, I just want to be prepared for the worse and when everyone around me is thinking I'm surviving, it's a little hard" I said

"Understandable, but you also need to have hope." she said to me, wanting to add a positive energy to my life.

"I had hope but now I know that I need to get my affairs in order." I explained

"Well…I'm here for you…as much as I don't act like it, I am" she said, leaning in for a hug.

"Thank you" I said as I hugged her goodbye.

For once in our short relationship, I felt truly close to Vera, she opened her hard shell, allowing me to see the true Vera. It was nice to have another person in my corner, not a family member or one of Henry's coworkers. She didn't need to be nice to me, but she chose to. She chose to support me without obligation.

~

Keeping my life in order became increasingly more difficult as my cancer advanced. I was drained of all my strength to be able to do anything. Everyone tells you to just go one with your day as normal, but no one ever tells you how much it takes to actually go through a normal day without pain or nausea or anxiety. I lost my ability to sew after my brain surgery, my drivers license was medically revoked, I was barely above to get to the zoo. I felt like it was losing everything that made me happy. Cancer began to take all of my joy and happiness in this world.

Henry was always working to support our little family, Daisy was either at school or the zoo, and my dad was still working full time even though he did move to New York to be closer. I was always alone; I never felt so isolated.

It was like being trapped in a bubble, separated from the world I once knew. Each day felt like a battle, not just against the illness ravaging my body, but against the loneliness and isolation that accompanied it. Everyone offered their support from afar, but the physical distance only accentuated the emotional void. Despite all of the support I had surrounding me, I still was unable to feel any ounce of happiness.

Simple pleasures became distant memories, replaced by the relentless cycle of treatments and doctor's appointments.

Chapter 17

I had to stay home to recover from brain surgery while Henry was always working. I had my dad, but it felt so isolating to be home instead of out exploring my new life. While I understood the necessity for him to go to work, it's challenging to be alone during the day, especially when I was dealing with such fatigue and discomfort. However, I tried to stay positive by focusing on my healing journey and finding solace in smallest of comforts. Whether it was reading a book, watching a comforting movie, or simply resting, I made sure to prioritize self-care and give myself the time and space I need to recover fully. Knowing my husband supported me and is there for me when he returns home gives me strength and motivation to keep pushing forward.

Worried I may scurry out of the house, Henry said, "Okay so I'm going to work, and you need to stay home... please"

He knew I was so determined to go back to the zoo, and I would do anything to get back to normal. While that is all I wanted, I had no strength left in me to get out of bed.

I assured him, "I will, I promise, I don't think I can find the strength to get up to go downstairs, let alone going out"

"Do you need me to stay home?" He asked me, not believing I'll actually stay home.

"No no no, go to work I will be fine, Daisy will be stopping by later and I'll have her help me" I said.

"Are you sure? I can take another day if you need" he pressed

"No Henry! Go to work!" I yelled

"Ok ok! Please be careful and let me know if you need anything." He said to me.

"I will, I promise... I love you" I repeated

"I love you too" he said

As my husband kissed me goodbye and headed off to work, I couldn't shake the sense of helplessness that washed over me. Crawling back into bed, I battled with the frustration of my own weakness, knowing I had no choice but to succumb to it. Every ounce of strength I possessed was consumed by the simple act of staying alive, confined to the stillness of my bed. Despite my longing for independence, I found myself trapped in a cycle of reliance, yearning for the day when I could reclaim control over my own body and destiny.

"Oh Menaaaa! I'm here to help!" I heard a loud voice come from the front door.

"I'm upstairs" I faintly yelled

"Hey, how ya feeling?" Daisy asked perky as ever.

"Like I got hit by a bus and then the bus backed up onto me again and again." I said

"Oh ok... well, I'm here to make your day better!" She replied

"Great…" I said

I just wanted to go to sleep but I know Daisy would never allow that. Daisy filled me in on all I was missing out on.

"How's the zoo?" I asked

"Good! Everyone's fed, happy, and safe!" She exclaimed

"They miss you though"

As I laughed at the thought of animals sensing my absence, memories of my college days flooded back, reminding me of the incredible abilities of our furry friends. I remembered learning about how animals could detect tumors by their distinct scent, a fact that always amazed me. Realizing every time I visited the zoo, they could likely smell my presence, I felt an overwhelming sense of both sadness and comfort. I've always been there for those animals, and hearing Daisy mention they missed me stirred up a mix of emotions. It made me sad to think about leaving them behind, but also reassured me my impact on their lives wouldn't be forgotten, even when I'm no longer around. Seems stupid with them being animals but they are so much more complex than what most people believe.

"I think we should offer free cancer screenings" Daisy suggested

"Can you just get me some soup?" I said faintly, dismissing her idea.

Knowing it would open up a world of lawsuits and problems, I thought it was a bad idea. But an ounce of me thought it kind of was a good idea…for a movie.

"It's a great idea!" She said

"Soup!" I yelled

"Ok ok! Just think about it though" she said as she walked downstairs.

As I dozed off, Daisy danced around the kitchen to make soup. By the time I woke up, she had already settled in front of the TV, enjoying the soup she had prepared for me. Watching her, I couldn't help but laugh at the simplicity of babysitting a cancer patient – all I seemed to do was sleep.

"Hey, what happened to my soup?" I asked as I slowly walked down the stairs.

"Oh… I uhh..." she said, startled

"You ate it?" I asked

"No, absolutely not! Someone came in and stole it!" She claimed

"Oh really?!" I laughed as I planted myself on the couch.

"Yes! I had to fight them off, it was very heroine" she said in a confident manner

We sat on the couch watching the daytime shows that no one else watched because everyone is busy at work or living their own lives. All while I sit at home, wasting away to a horrible death.

~

Despite the exhaustion weighing me down, there was a burning desire within me to dance, if only for a moment, to reclaim a sense of normalcy in the midst of battling cancer. It was more than just movement; it was a yearning to reconnect with the vibrant spirit I once possessed. With each step, I felt Philomena, the person I used to be, slowly returning. It was a fleeting escape from the harsh reality of illness, a brief respite where I could lose myself in the rhythm and let the music wash away the pain, if only for a little while.

Step by step, I felt Philomena come back.

As the music filled the room, Daisy caught the contagious energy, joining me in a spontaneous dance. Despite the weight of the situation, her youthful exuberance brought a spark of joy to the moment.

Together, we moved with a carefree abandon, laughing and twirling as if we were teenagers again. In her presence, the heaviness of my illness momentarily lifted, replaced by the lightness of shared laughter and youthful spirit. It was a reminder that even in the darkest times, moments of pure joy and connection could still be found.

"So, I'll take that soup when you get a chance" I said

I fell into the couch from exhaustion, Feeling as light as ever.

"Oh, ok I'll go do that!" Daisy said, out of breath from our little dance moment.

"Thank you" I said "So I'm thinking I'm going to head back to the zoo next week"

"No girl, take a break!" Daisy replied

"No, it's fine, I'll be fine" I assured her.

"Seriously, the last time you were there you almost died" Daisy said in a concerned tone.

She didn't want the responsibility of my health in her hands. I gave her the biggest scare of her life after I passed out in her car.

"I think your being a bit dramatic" I laughed

"No, I'm not, I can't lose you, almost losing you was the worst feeling in the world" Daisy responded Realizing she was making it about herself she cut herself off. Daisy has never been put in this situation so everything, including conversations, were new to her. She didn't want to make me feel uncomfortable or insulted so she constantly walked on eggshells when it came to anything she said.

"I'm sorry…" she said

"It's not your fault… I just… need to get back to whatever normal life I have." I replied

She went on to make soup and I headed back to bed. On a typical day, I slept for 14 hours and stayed in bed for the other 10. Only waking up or leaving my bed to go to the bathroom or vomit. I knew my time was dwindling and I was getting weaker by the day. I also knew I needed to get my affairs in order sooner rather than later.

Henry came home to find me asleep yet again. I felt extremely nauseated from the soup I ate, regretting it with each small movement I made.

"Leave me alone" I said as I laid in bed

"I can't, you need to take your medication" he said holding a cup of pills

"What's the point?" I said

I pulled the sheets up, trying to get him to go away so I could fall back asleep.

"They will make you feel better!" he assured me.

"No, they won't... they never do" I argued

"Okay well they're going to help you" he replied

I continued to refuse my meds and he became increasingly frustrated by my reluctance.

"What? Move my timeline by a few weeks?" I said

"What is your problem?" He slowly realized he wasn't going to win the argument.

He placed the medications on the nightstand and began to walk away.

"I'm not having this conversation right now, I'm the one dying, not you! So, I need you to stop acting like we are doing this together because we are not!" I yelled before he left the room.

Despite Henry's insistence, I refused to take my medications. The pills became a daily reminder of my illness, a bitter pill to swallow both literally and figuratively. Yet, I knew deep down that they were essential for my well-being, a lifeline in the battle against cancer. It was a constant internal struggle, wavering between the desire to defy the disease and the need to heed medical advice. His unwavering support and concern only added to the conflict, a constant reminder of the importance of prioritizing my health even when every fiber of my being rebelled against it.

Henry crawled into bed, exhausted from work as well as arguing with me. As he joined me in bed, I reminded him of all of the things I need to do to prepare for my death.

"We have a meeting with a lawyer tomorrow, he's coming here because I can't get out of bed long enough to leave the house. Therefore, you can wake me up when he's here, we will handle my will, and then I will get back to bed and you go back to work. Done!" I said to him

"You are the biggest pain in the ass!" He said, pulling the sheets I had taken from his side

"You'll remember that if I die tonight" I replied

"You won't even try to die tonight, you have too much of a need for control to die before figuring out where all of your shit goes!" He argued, despite our continuous disagreements, he turned the lights off while still reminding me that he loves me.

~

He knew me too well that I would never leave without knowing where all of my things were going. I wasn't materialistic in the slightest, but I wanted to know my future was in good hands. It's not like I had any kids or much family to pass on my belongings.

As the lawyer arrived at my doorstep to discuss my will, a wave of solemnity washed over me, confronting the harsh reality of my situation head-on. It was a necessary yet daunting task, facing the inevitability of my own mortality and the need to ensure my affairs were in order.

Sitting down with pen in hand, I felt a sense of gravity settle in the room, each word spoken carrying the weight of finality. Despite the discomfort of confronting such matters, there was a strange sense of peace in knowing that I was taking proactive steps to provide for my loved ones even after I was gone.

I found myself uneasy with the lawyer's overly cheerful vibe. His oddly cheerful demeanor felt contradicting to his career and the only reason he was sitting in my living room. It felt discordant with the gravity of the situation, leaving me feeling unsettled and misunderstood. While I appreciated his attempt to lighten the mood, I couldn't shake the feeling he was trivializing the seriousness of the matter at hand. His bubbly energy clashed with my own somber mood, creating a sense of dissonance that made it difficult to fully engage in the conversation.

"Good morning" the lawyer said cheerfully

"Hi so I'm going to be honest, I need to make this quick because I don't want to be doing this, but I have to because I am dying."

I cut him off from his basic introduction he says to every client he has.

"Okay well we won't be long; your husband has informed me you did some pre-planning" he replied

"I did, I just need to make it official" I said

"Well, that's my job" he laughed

"Good so let's get this over with" I said, keeping my emotions in check, not feeding into his bubbly behavior.

"I'm sorry… she just hasn't really accepted this whole situation" my husband interjected

"It's okay. I see it many times" the lawyer said to Henry.

"Great, so let's focus!" I responded

"I have no children, my husband is pretty much the only family I have, I'm not even from New York so it's not like I'm leaving much here. This should make your job easy" I explained as I watched him pull piles of unorganized paperwork in his worn-down briefcase.

"She just wants to make sure her zoo is in line" Henry said

"Your zoo?" He asked, pausing his paper search

"Yes, my zoo!" I said "I need my zoo to be in the right hands"

"Have you thought about selling it?" He asked

"No no, it's staying in the family. I need the title to go to my husband. my niece, Daisy, will run the place.

"Umm yea I think that's it!" I said, trying to quickly wrap everything up.

"Okay great we will put the title to Henry Williams and Daisy Williams will be the…" the lawyer jotted down

"CEO, Daisy will be the CEO" I finished his sentence

"I don't think that's how that works" Henry replied

"Well, that's how I'm making it work" I said

"Will do!" The lawyer smiled "So anything else?"

"I have a lot of shoes; they should go to Daisy as well" I said "just give my wardrobe to Daisy. My neighbor always loved my glass collection… give it to her"

"What's her name?" He asked

I asked Henry for his secretary's full name as I never took the time to learn it.

"Vera Sevnicks" he replied

"Sevnicks… Vera" I repeated,

I was staring at the bird feeder, watching all of the birds pass through.

"Great!" Henry said, "Okay I think that's it?"

"Are you sure?" The lawyer said trying to get my attention

"Yes, I told you, I have nothing important so yes I need these things to go to the right place" I replied in a short manner.

All I wanted to do was to go back to bed so I tried to push the lawyer out.

"Okay, I just need a couple of signatures from you and then I will be on my way!" The lawyer responded

"How long will this take to be official?" I asked

"Officially it can take up to a year-" he explained

"I don't have a year left" I stopped him

"Ya haven't let me finish." He said "as long as I have your signature then everything is set in stone from here on out"

"Okay, perfect, well you have a great day and feel free to send a copy to my husband when I'm gone!" I said

I quickly got up to guide him to the door, he tried to continue the conversation, but I slammed the door on him without giving him a chance to finish.

"You can be a little nicer" Henry said from the living room

"He wasn't the nicest" I argued

"Yes, he was! You were being the rude one" he replied

"Pardon me for being a little less than enthusiastic about dying at the grand old age of 24." I said as I walked up stairs to head back to bed.

"I understand…" I heard him say from a distance.

"No, Henry, you don't" I said as I stood at the foot of the stairs.

I watched him pour his heart out to him. Finally showing his emotions for once.

"Do you think I want this? You think I want to lose my first love this quickly?" He yelled

"Henry… I don't want to die" I said as tears welled in my eyes.

I ran to him, hugging him as we sat on the couch.

"I know you don't, and I don't want you to die. But you are and I am going to lose you. I don't know what I'm going to do without you, but I have you now and I need to focus on now. Because if I focus on the future then I won't be able to keep myself together. You're focusing on the future, yet you have no future! So, stop this bullshit of dying and live. Just live for however long you have!" He explained in a passionate tone, comforting me.

I paused, again looking out the window at the birds.

"Thank you" I replied

"For what?" He asked

"I don't know, just thank you for being here and dealing with me" I said through my sobs

"I'm not dealing with you" he laughed

"But you are, I've been so rude and dramatic to you, and you just take it! I'm sorry and I love you so much!" I replied

"I love you too and I will always love you forever and ever" he said

He began to rub my back as we stayed nestled on the couch, both of us watching the birds feeding on the mix.

Accepting the reality of my own mortality has always been a daunting task, one that I still struggle with today. It feels as though everyone around me is coming to terms with my impending death, yet I remain stuck in a state of denial, unable to fully grasp the gravity of the situation. It's a lonely feeling, being left behind in my own journey towards the inevitable. While others may offer words of comfort and support, ultimately, I am the one who must confront the harsh reality of my mortality, a journey I am still navigating with uncertainty and fear.

Chapter 18

Summoning all my strength, I decided to make possibly one last visit to the zoo. I knew I probably wouldn't have much longer. I remember when my mom was dying, she could sense her body giving way. Now as I am dying myself, I understand how it feels to know your time is limited. It was weird but I felt comforted in knowing I was dying. I was prepared, ready for my next stage. I knew my life was in order and I was ready to die, something I never though I'd say.

As I strolled through the familiar paths, I found myself captivated by the scenes unfolding around me. Children laughed and played, parents chased after them with fond exasperation, and elderly couples shared quiet moments feeding the birds. The monkeys swung gracefully from tree to tree, their agility a testament to the beauty of life's simple pleasures. In the distance, the wolves howled in harmony with the hawks soaring overhead, while the pandas frolicked amongst the bamboo, their playful antics a reminder of the joy found in the present moment. And as the majestic elephants performed their water show with graceful trunks, I couldn't help but feel a sense of peace wash over me, grateful for the opportunity to witness the beauty of life in all its forms one last time. I witnessed all of this every time I went to the zoo but this time, it felt different. I knew I was getting weaker, and my body was hinting to me that I was losing my battle.

These animals were so full of life while I had a mere few months left. I wasn't scared, more so angry. I was angry that I was going to be missing out on so much and leaving this world so soon. While it was infuriated, I still was not scared of death. I accepted death in a way, just a little bit. I wasn't scared of death, I was scared of leaving all of this behind. I was not ready to let everything go.

"You're here, how are you feeling?" Daisy asked me as she came up from behind me.

"I'm okay, I'm doing okay" I said sitting on a bench in front of the sea lion enclosure.

"That's good!" Daisy replied

"How's everything been" I asked

"Good. Oh! The lion had her cubs!" She responded excitedly

"Oh, that's good, I'll have to stop by" I said in a very monotone tone.

She asked me as if she could sense my somber feeling. "What's wrong?"

"What do you mean?" I asked, trying to shake my feeling of depression.

"You were so excited to find out she was expecting cubs and now you are acting like it's just another day" she replied

"Nothings wrong, I'm just as happy as I was when I found out." I assured her, walking to my office.

I left her to work on other things, trying to get her to leave me alone. I was exhausted from constantly having people ask me the same questions and having the same 'cancer conversations' every time.

"Morning Philomena" my accounts manager said to me as I walked into the room

"Don't say anything" I replied

"Wasn't planning on it?" She replied, going back to her paperwork.

"Good, do you have those budget plans for next quarter?" I asked her

"How are you feeling?" She asked

"See that's what I mean, don't ask!" I said, annoyed as ever.

"Will do" she stopped herself from speaking anymore.

I knew she would probably mention how sickly I looked, just like everyone else. I had lost so much weight, and I gave up on wearing a wig. Henry gave me a plethora of different head scarves. It became a hobby to match different scarves with different outfits. I had fun finding a matching outfits, it gave me a sense of style in something that was so depressing.

Daisy walked up to the offices. She was used to my avoidant behavior. I didn't want to talk to anyone about my cancer because it was just a reminder I could have as little as a month left to live. My cancer was progressing fast, and I didn't have the strength to explain it to everyone. I just wanted to act as though everything was normal.

"Well, she's back I can tell" the accounts manager said

"Have you ever heard of a premortem surge" Daisy asked, worried I was on my way out, sooner rather than later.

"She's not there, that's for people who are not even able to get out of bed or recognize anything" she replied, assuring Daisy I was not in that situation.

"That's true…" Daisy said

She watched me on my computer, doing as much work as I possibly could. I was rigorously typing while ignoring everything around me.

"Well, I have to run to the bank and then I'll be back, want a coffee?" The accounts manager replied, grabbing her keys and coat, trying to deescalate the situation.

"Iced latte with cinnamon!" Daisy replied

~

Henry was at work. Busy distracting himself from the thought of becoming a young widow.

"Good morning Mr. Williams" Vera said as he came in

He was late because he had to clean my vomit up from the sheets that had been sitting there since 4am, I didn't want wake him, so he didn't notice until we woke up. I cleaned most of it, but Henry had to handle the rest before leaving for work.

"Morning, thank you for the coffee!" Henry replied

"No problem, how's Philomena?" She asked

"She's doing okay, she's actually at the zoo today!" He said with a smile on his face.

I haven't been out of the house besides chemo, so everyone saw me at the zoo as a big triumph for me. I felt as though they were treating me like a child who just learned to potty train.

"That's great!" Vera said

"Yea, I can't keep up with when she's good when she's not. She's just never on one page." Henry laughed

"Oh, I Get that, she's crazy!" She replied

"I don't know what I'm going to do when she's gone" Henry said in a somber voice

"You'll get through it…" she comforted him

"Easier said than done" he said as he got all of his things on his desk.

"You never told me how you guys met?" She asked, genuinely curious.

"We met in high school, in Economics class." he explained "I remember we did our final project together. We had to create a business. Completely follow through with a proposal, budget, the whole gig. I didn't really care for it, but she loved it, so I let her do the whole project. She was so mad after a while because I did nothing, but I made up some lie my parents needed me home right after school. One day she just told me that she would come over to work on the project and I told my parents a girl was coming over. They freaked out and were so excited thinking we were dating and it kind of turned into a date somehow."

"That's cute, so your parents' kind of hooked you two up" she replied

"I guess so, it took us a while to fully understand what we were but eventually she asked me out and said, 'since everyone else thinks we're dating, why don't we just do it' and we went to the State theater and watched the Swan Lake ballet." He continued

"The ballet?" She smirked

"Yea she loved it, but I fell asleep halfway through" he laughed

"Your horrible" she said as she threw a stack of papers onto his desk

"I know I know, but it was just so boring… but what I would do to go back to that day again…" he said, thinking back to that day.

"Well let's go talk to study council about these trips they have planned" Henry said

"What's their plan for money?" Vera asked

"No clue" he said as they walked down the hall to the conference room.

The student council had planned for a trip to the science museum and the students also had other plans.

They all sat at the round top table, all of the students talking about the different ideas they had for the upcoming year. This was a big meeting for them as they were planning for the end of the year.

"So, we need your permission obviously, but we wanted to do something for your wife" the student council president explained further, "We know you're going through a lot right now and us and the entire school want to show our support for you and Mrs. Williams."

"I- I'm honored" Henry said as Vera rubbed his back, comforting him knowing he would most likely get emotional.

"We would love to show our support at a track and field meet. We are raising money for shirts, money for the zoo, and we are planning for the whole school to attend" the president explained

"I just don't know what to say…" Henry said as tears welled in Vera's eyes. "Thank you…"

"BUT we don't want her to know so could you keep it a secret?" Another student added

"Yes, but I'm going to be honest with you guys…she is not well" he interjected

"Set a date and she will be there" Vera interjected

"Great! We are looking forward to it!" The students said excitedly.

He pulled Vera to the outside in the hallway, he wanted to have Vera face the reality that I was probably not going to make it.

"Why did you agree to that?" Henry said

"Because she's family and they want to do something do for family" Vera said

"Yea but what if she doesn't make it" Henry asked

"Henry… Just let them do it…" Vera argued

"Fine… just be prepared to have that conversation with them because I'm not explaining to them that she's dead!" he said as he stormed off.

Vera stayed in the meeting and Henry left as the science discussion was over. He locked himself into his office and cried for the first time. Henry doesn't cry, he locks his emotions up tight and never lets anyone see it. Including me. You know the cancer was winning when it finally gets Henry to cry.

~

I went home early from the zoo and went to bed.
But I couldn't fall asleep, so I waited for Henry to come
home so he could cook dinner. It was weird to feel an
appetite because I couldn't eat without throwing up. I just
was so scared to feel good because I wasn't sure what it
meant.

An onset of bone pain gripped me relentlessly, a
constant throbbing ache that seemed to seep into every
fiber of my being. As I lay in bed, the torment of each
movement echoed through my body, making sleep an
elusive dream. Every shift in position sent waves of
agony coursing through me, leaving me trapped in a state
of restless discomfort. The darkness of the night only
magnified the intensity of the pain, amplifying my sense
of isolation and despair. Hours stretched on endlessly as
I yearned for relief, longing for the respite of sleep to
grant me even a moment's reprieve from the relentless
torment of my bones.

In the midst of my suffering, my husband's support
was a beacon of comfort amidst the darkness. With a
gentle touch and a reassuring voice, he offered me

medication to ease the pain, his presence a source of solace in the midst of my turmoil. His unwavering dedication to my well-being gave me strength to endure, reminding me I was not facing this battle alone. With each tender gesture, he promised his commitment to walk beside me through the darkest of nights, offering both physical reprieve and unwavering support as we navigated this journey together.

Struggling with the constant waves of nausea, pain, and fatigue, I found myself unable to muster the courage to broach the topic of stopping chemotherapy with Henry. Each day, the burden of these symptoms, compounded by the effects of both the treatment and the cancer itself, grew heavier. It became increasingly clear to me my terminal prognosis offered little hope of change, and the continued ordeal of chemotherapy only served to prolong my suffering. I longed for a dignified end, to pass away as myself rather than confined to a hospital bed or reduced to a state of unawareness. It was a difficult realization, but one that I knew I needed to confront for the sake of my own peace and dignity.

Chapter 19

I needed to find the right time to talk to Henry but there just never seemed to be an appropriate time to tell your husband that you want to end your treatment and die.

"Hey Henry, I'm going to get dinner tonight so maybe come home early?" I said to him as he left for work.

This man never made it home on time, so it was nearly impossible to plan anything at night.

"Yea I'll sneak out early, what are we having?" He asked.

"Not sure yet, it'll be a surprise" I smiled

"Ok…No fish, I'm still paying for the fish and chips from a few weeks ago" he added

"Wasn't planning on it" I laughed remembering when his fish and chips turned him into a chemo patient for a night.

"Great! See you tonight" He kissed me goodbye and left for work.

I decided to go back to bed and find something for dinner before I fell asleep. My bone pain was still unbearable, but I didn't want to become so drugged up that I couldn't function, so I just dealt with it.

"Philomena?" I heard a distant voice coming from downstairs.

I was awoken from my nap to my dad visiting, maybe for the last time. I couldn't get out of bed, so I had him come upstairs to my little cancer throne.

"How are you feeling sweetie?" He asked as he creaked the door open, peering in.

"I'm doing ok" I replied, welcoming him into the room.

He leaned in to hug me, but I stopped him before. "Please don't hug me…" I said as I grabbed him hand. "I'm sorry… I just am in so much pain that I can't be touched…" I added

"Oh baby…" he said, holding back tears from seeing me in such agony.

"It's okay, I know it's from my medications so it's not a bad sign" I assured him

"Can't they change your medications?" He asked me.

"I don't think so, it's for my white blood cells which are too low, so I guess this is just my bones making white blood cells" I replied

"Okay… so it's helping your immune system?" he asked

"Yes exactly" I said

He continued, "Is this a good sign for your prognosis?"

"Dad… you know I'm not getting out of this" I said to him

"You don't know that… if your immune system is stronger then maybe it could fight the cancer as well as the chemo and radiation." He said, as he began to cry.

He continued to argue with me trying to help me find a way out of this. When in reality, I had no way out and I needed him to understand this.

"Philomena do not think like that" he argued passionately

"It's a lose, lose situation, chemo kills my white blood cells, this pegfilgrastim or whatever gives me my white blood cells, then I'm in pain. If I want to not be in pain, then I could get sick and die. My white blood cells help my cancer but the chemo which also helps my cancer kills my blood cells. Make it make sense!" I explained, now crying from having such a difficult conversation with my dad, I wasn't even sure if I made sense to myself.

He held my hand, sitting on the side of the bed with me. "You can do this, you are so damn strong, and I know you can get through this" he said

I quickly tried to change the conversation, knowing he wouldn't give up, "Can you grab some chicken broth from downstairs?" I asked him

"Sure…" he felt defeated, he nursed my mom for so long before she passed, and he was facing that same searing pain he felt before.

He remembered how much pain her death caused him and now he has to go through it all over again.

He asked, "Why can't we talk about this?"

"Because this is my battle" I argued knowing he had no idea how I felt.

"I lost your mother, I don't want to lose my only daughter too" he replied, he refused to leave my side without talking about what was going on.

While all I wanted to do was sleep and he wanted to argue about my decision to end treatment and face death in my own way.

"I'm not mom…mom caused her death by doing stupid things like smoking and drinking her liver away. I didn't choose this; I did everything right and yet I'll still be dead at 24!" I argued, exhausted from the conversation.

"Chicken broth…and noodles?" He said walking towards the door, knowing he's about to lose his daughter.

"No, I'll throw them up" I replied

"You should really try and get more calories" he said before leaving

"It's not worth it, it'll just come back up along with the chicken broth…" I explained.

"Okay I'll be back" he said as he walked to the door "love you honey bun"

"I love you too dad" he

He went and warmed my soup, then we watched daytime soap operas for a while when I realized I forgot about dinner, being so exhausted and in pain, I didn't feel like I had the strength to cook a full dinner.

"Wait! Can you cook dinner? I completely forgot that I told Henry I would have dinner ready for when he got home" I asked him before he headed home.

"What are we thinking, pasta, hamburgers, chicken cordon bleu?" He asked me with a smile on his face.

"Spaghetti and meatballs sound so good!" I replied

"It'll be ready before he even leaves the office" he smiled

"You are amazing!" I said as I gently hugged him

My dad took my entire kitchen and turned it into a warm, intimate setting for a lovely dinner. The whole room was filled with the smell of fresh garlic, warm baked bread, and a sense of Italy in my own home.

The clock was hitting 3:30 and Henry would be home before five. I didn't want my dad to be here for the conversation I was going to have with my husband, so I rushed him out before. My dad had a light feeling thinking we were having an intimate night together as husband and wife. I didn't want to dampen his spirits, so I went along with it, maybe I was slightly hoping for that to actually be true.

My dad left and I anxiously waited for Henry to get home from work. I wanted to finally tell him I needed to stop treatments, but I knew he would have pushback. I had a pit in my stomach as I waited for him.

I dreaded the conversation but seeing my chemo not doing anything but hurt me, made me hope for a breath of fresh air after this conversation.

~

Henry made it home with 10 minutes to spare and he seemed exhausted from a long day's work. He walked into the kitchen, following the smell of the magnificent tomato sauce simmering on the stove. I watched him explore all of the food, shocked I would have the strength to do all of it. I stopped his praise to explain my dad's talents that I definitely did not inherit.

"How was work?" I asked as I kissed him

"Not too bad, kids these days are just insane, like I can't imagine what my parents would do if I acted like some of these kids!" He replied, unable to imagine the conversation I was about to have with him.

"Yea times have definitely changed" I said, hesitating on bringing up what I needed to. "I need to talk to you and get your advice on something" I paused

"Looking to finally sell the zoo?" He laughed as he played a dish of spaghetti

"No Henry…" I said, in an opposite tone

"I'm just joking" he smiled "what's going on?"

He came over to the kitchen table with two plates. I stared at it seeing that he still had confidence in my being able to eat.

"I want to stop treatment" I said bluntly.

He stopped and stared, not saying anything for a minute. The last thing he imagined thinking about when ending a busy day at work was his wife's decision to die. He knew deep down it was my decision but felt the need to take control.

"No" he replied

"Henry-" I said, trying to contain my emotions

"No Philomena, that is not an option. You can't just throw the towel in because your doctors are giving you statistics that don't mean anything!" He replied, tears streaming down his face.

"I'm dying Henry, and my body can't take anymore of this!" I replied,

"Do you really understand what you are saying?" he asked me, thinking I was just being dramatic.

"Yes, I understand I am dying, and chemo is just making it worse. I want to die without being so sick I can't recognize you or just lay in bed waiting to die in pain and agony. I'm in so much pain and I want to be able to die without suffering" I explained.

We sat at the kitchen table, staring into each other's eyes, both filled with tears. Holding hands from across. We both forgot the food was sitting there among us.

"Chemo isn't working, is it?" He asked, pulling back

"No, it's not, my cancer is not getting any better. It won Henry… I'm done…" I replied, somberly

As his arms wrapped around me, I felt the weight of his understanding and acceptance. It was a comforting reassurance to know I wasn't alone in this choice, that someone stood by me in solidarity, recognizing the gravity of my decision and respecting my autonomy.

With his embrace, I found strength in knowing that even amidst uncertainty, I had someone who believed in me and supported my journey ahead onto my next story.

Feeling the weight of mounting bills and the strain on my family, I realized the stark reality: my doctors were pushing treatments primarily for financial gain. It was a difficult truth to face, knowing my suffering was not just physical but also financial, burdening those I love. The decision to halt treatment wasn't solely about my own pain but also about sparing my family from further financial hardship. Despite the guilt of feeling selfish, I understood prolonging my suffering with ineffective treatments was no longer justifiable. It was time to prioritize peace and hav what ability of letting go, even amidst the uncertainty that lay ahead.

I needed Henry to understand my decision, but accepting my impending death was incredibly hard for him. Despite the support he showed me during my final days, he couldn't bring himself to let me go. It was my time, though. My days and nights were spent in bed, either asleep or in pain. All I wanted was for it to end, but Henry wished for just a few more weeks. I didn't have a few more weeks in me. Day by day, I could feel my body giving out. Through each moment, Henry stayed by my side.

It's strange how your body tells you when it's time. Towards the end, I felt an overwhelming sense of calm. It was as if my body, in sync with my brain, was preparing me for the inevitable. Henry stood by me until the very last moment. My final sight was his face, flooded with tears, as he gently whispered that it was okay to let go. In that moment, surrounded by love and acceptance, I felt a profound peace, knowing I was not alone and that my journey was coming to its natural end.

As my breaths grew shallow, I could feel the weight of the world lifting from my shoulders. Memories of our life together, from our first meeting to this final farewell, played like a beautiful montage in my mind. I thought of the zoo, the sanctuary we built, and the laughter of children and families that would continue to echo within its walls. I hoped Henry would find comfort in those memories and the legacy we created. My last thoughts were of gratitude—for the love we shared, for the life I lived, and for the peaceful transition I was blessed with. With one final breath, I let go, embraced by the calmly Heaven that had been waiting for me.

Chapter 20

Henry sat in the stillness of the empty brownstone, the memories of his wedding day flickered vividly in his mind, each moment etched with bittersweet clarity. The joy of their first dance enveloped him, a fleeting respite from the weight of grief had settled upon his shoulders.

Lost in reverie, he hardly noticed the gentle knock on the door, a subtle interruption to the solitude that now defined his existence.

"Mind if I come in?" His father-in-law said in a solemn tone

"No, not at all" he said "I have makers mark or there's Mena's pinot in the cabinet"

"I'm okay, I have to drive" he replied

"How are you holding up?" He asked

Henry sat in my chair near the window that faced the birds. As all of the memories of our time together raced through his mind, he asked my dad quietly, "Do you remember our wedding?"

"Yes, I remember you both couldn't agree on the flowers to chose" he laughed

"We ended up with red roses, the first of many disagreements I would lose" Henry added "It always needed to be her way"

"It's funny because she always did get her way... down to her death, down to her last breath" he said

~

Henry sat by the window of the living room, his gaze fixed on the lively scene unfolding outside: children playing in the street, birds flocking to the feeder. As he prepared to head to the funeral, a flash of crimson caught his eye—a cardinal, perched delicately amid a bed of roses. A soft smile tugged at his lips as he followed the bird's graceful flight into the bright blue sky.

Despite the emptiness weighing heavily in his heart, he found a sense of peace in the presence of the cardinal, a silent reminder of a love that transcended past earthly bounds. In that moment, he knew I would always be by his side, even if only in the form of a gentle creature.

Henry made sure to allow for a peaceful passing. He knew I was going, following all of my requests to die in my own way. No hospitals, no tubes, or wires. I had no control of my life, but I had control of my death. Warm blankets, fluffy pillows, the graceful hand of my husband stroking my head. The window cracked open to allow the breeze of the spring air, the birds chirping away in a solemn melody. Henry kept me warm; we laid in bed together just like every other day.

My dad lost his only girl. He held the thought of his only family being reunited again. While we didn't get along at all, really, God brought us back together. My mom and I were able to reignite our friendship from beyond this light.

At the great age of 48, he found himself forced to pick up the pieces of his shattered life and carry on alone. Despite the immense burden of grief and loss, he persevered and walked with his head held high, refusing to succumb to despair. With every step forward, he confronted the stark reality of his solitude, grappling with the absence of his entire family, however small it may have been. The loss of his only daughter cut him to the core, leaving a void which seemed impossible to fill. Yet, within the depths of his sorrow, he drew strength from the memories of his beloved child. In the face of adversity, he dared to believe he could rebuild his life, piece by fragile piece, and forge a new path illuminated by courage and hope.

My dad and Henry shared a bond forged in loss, both grappling with the absence of the one who brought light and joy into their lives. United by grief, they found comfort in each other's company, navigating the turbulent seas of sorrow together. Their connection transcended words, a silent understanding born from shared experiences of longing and heartache. In each other's presence, they found fleeting moments of reassurance, reminders of the love they had lost and the strength they carried within. Despite the shadows that lingered, they clung to the hope that, together, they could weather the storm and find glimpses of sunshine amidst the darkness.

Daisy, with her youthful vigor and unyielding determination, became the lifeline of the zoo, tirelessly working to ensure its prosperity and preserving my legacy even after my passing. Despite her young age, she possessed a remarkable ability to captivate visitors and breathe new vitality into the sanctuary for each of its animals. Every day, she seemed to possess an innate connection with the animals, nurturing their well-being and fostering an environment where they could thrive.

With boundless energy and a passion for conservation, Daisy transformed the zoo into a haven of wonder and excitement, drawing in crowds with her innovative ideas and unwavering commitment to the welfare of every creature under her care. In her hands, my dream continued to flourish, a testament to her unwavering dedication and the enduring spirit of the legacy we built together.

My Henry was my rock, comforting me as I prepared to embark on my final journey. The realization I couldn't bring him along by my side shattered me, knowing our bond would be confined to this life. As I crossed the threshold into the unknown, leaving him behind weighed heavily on my soul. Even as I journeyed onwards to Heaven, without him physically present, I took comfort in the knowledge that his love would continue to guide me, making the transition less daunting. In their unwavering presence, I found peace, knowing I was not alone as I embraced what lay ahead.

A part of me yearned for Henry to find peace and move forward. Though the thought of him carrying on without me was bittersweet, I knew clinging to my memory would only burden him with unnecessary grief. I wanted him to embrace life's beauty once again, to find joy in the simple pleasures, and to discover new paths illuminated by hope and possibility. Though my absence would leave an irreplaceable void in his heart, I wished for him to cherish our memories while opening his heart to the promise of tomorrow. Watching him forge ahead, carrying my love within him, would have brought me a sense of peace as I journeyed onwards.

Henry may be my ending… but I am not his….

~

In the end, dying from cancer was a deeply personal journey, marked by moments of pain, fear, and sadness, but also by moments of love, connection, and unexpected grace. It was a journey that ultimately led me to confront the fragility of life and the importance of finding peace and acceptance in the face of adversity.

Now, from the vantage point beyond life's veil, I see the truth in his words. Death, while daunting, offered respite from the ceaseless torment of illness. In my final moments, I found solace in the release from suffering, understanding sometimes, peace lies not in the fight against mortality, but in the acceptance of its inevitable embrace.

Cancer was a relentless foe, one I wouldn't wish upon anyone, not even my worst enemy. No one chooses to be ill; I certainly didn't. I struggled to comprehend why fate singled me out for such a vicious affliction. How could such a benevolent God allow a 24-year-old to endure such a harrowing demise? Henry's words, however, rang true: dying was, indeed, the easier part.

Glossary

Brownstone- Fairly unique to New York and other cities, row homes in popular among middle class families in the 19th century.

Fibroadenoma- A benign, solid lump in the breast, typically, painless.

Hamartomas- Benign clump of cells and tissue found in various parts of the body

Acerbic- Sharp or bitter in tone

Triple negative breast cancer- Tumor that tests negative for estrogen, progesterone, and HER2

Progesterone hormone- Steroid, sex hormone found in ovaries and testes, as well as being secreted from the adrenal glands

Estrogen- Specific to women; secretes from adrenal
glands and helps regulate normal sexual and
reproductive development

Human epidermal growth factor receptor 2 (HER2)-
Aids in controlling cell growth and cell division

Lumpectomy- Surgery to remove cancer cells in the
breast while preserving healthy breast tissue

Mastectomy- Surgery to remove both cancer and healthy
breast tissue to prevent the risk of tumors returning
in the future.

Mets- Secondary growth of tumors in other parts of the
body

Craniotomy- Small piece of the skull Is removed to
expose the brain, in order to remove a tumor or
solve other Issues in the brain

Parietal lobe- Section in the brain that controls senses and
pain

Pegfilgrastim- Injection to stimulate the production of
white blood cells

PEACE AMONG THE ANIMALS